"I spent two years suffering in ꜱilenᴄe ꜰrom debilitating anxiety. I would have given anything for a copy of *Mental Health Emergencies*. These illnesses affect every single person on the planet—whether it's you, your parents, your best friend, or your co-workers. Read it, and make this world a better place."

> **—Charlie Hoehn, author of** *Play It Away: A Workaholic's Cure for Anxiety*

"If we are going to truly tackle stigma and the barriers millions of Americans face when it comes to getting access to treatment, we need to start by equipping those on the front lines with the skills to recognize mental illness and direct people to the help they deserve. Nick Benas' book couldn't come at a better time as those of us involved in this cause search for new partners in the fight for better mental health in this country."

> **—Sean Scanlon, Connecticut State Representative**

"I have been supporting children between the ages of 9–12 for the past 12 years as a school counselor. Not only have I experienced years of anxiety growing up, I see it impacting the lives of our youth. Nick Benas' book will be a powerful tool for not only the children but for professional development."

> **—Paul Canestri, Middle School Counselor, Guilford, CT**

"As a Pastor and a Chaplain in the L.A. County Jails, this timely book is an indispensable tool for me to better understand and assist these friends. I hope it will inspire more to reach out to ones who desperately need to know there is someone who cares about them."

    —Chaplain Martin Wilson, Pastor of the Beverly Hills Persian Church

"Mental illness and military veterans have gone through several changes within the past decade and a half. Today, you see many veterans and veteran organizations not only speaking out in support of treatment for mental illness, but the civilian world as well. Veterans are no longer feeling as stigmatized by mental illness, but we still have a long way to go and this book will help."

    —Matt Bloom, LSW, Combat Veteran SGT USMC

"When most people think of "emergency," they immediately think of physical ailments. But the idea that all of us can be prepared to offer help for mental health emergency is both poignant and eye-opening. This book offers convenient heuristics that empower the reader to assist friends and loved ones when they need it most, while also surfacing the critical harbingers that signify when first aid may not be enough."

    —Matt Sitomer VP, Group Account Director VaynerMedia

"Nick Benas explains such simple and effective strategies to aid, assist, and provide the necessary resources for those struggling with mental health and substance use."

—**Brian Cuban, best-selling author of** *Shattered Image: My Triumph over Body Dysmorphic Disorder*

"If we are going to truly tackle stigma and the barriers millions of Americans face when it comes to getting access to treatment, we need to start by equipping those on the front lines with the skills to recognize mental illness and direct people to the help they deserve. Nick Benas' book couldn't come at a better time as those of us involved in this cause search for new partners in the fight for better mental health in this country."

—**Sean Scanlon, Connecticut State Representative**

"That social workers are employed in more and more libraries is evidence of the growing mental health crisis in our country. Mental Health Emergencies is a much needed resource for those of us without the luxury of a social worker on staff. Don't go to work without it!"

—**Anne Odom, Senior Library Assistant and Mediator**

MENTAL HEALTH EMERGENCIES

A First-Responder's Guide to Recognizing and Handling Mental Health Crises

NICK BENAS

AND

MICHELE HART, LCSW

Foreword by Ben Biddick, co-author of
Get Up: The Art of Perseverance

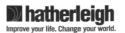
Improve your life. Change your world.

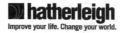
Improve your life. Change your world.

Hatherleigh Press is committed to preserving and protecting the natural resources of the earth. Environmentally responsible and sustainable practices are embraced within the company's mission statement.

Visit us at www.hatherleighpress.com and register online for free offers, discounts, special events, and more.

Mental Health Emergencies

Library of Congress Cataloging-in-Publication Data is available.
ISBN: 978-1-57826-674-6

DISCLAIMER

The information provided in this book is an information resource only, and is not intended for use as a diagnostic or treatment tool. It is meant to supplement, not replace, proper professional medical and mental health training. The authors have spent most of their professional career working in various positions in social services and mental health. This information is not intended for patient/consumer education, nor does it represent any patient/physician or provider-type relationship, and should not be used as a substitute for professional clinical diagnosis and/or treatment.

Please note that, as a first responder, you may be confronted with situations involving unique and uncontrollable environmental factors and accompanying risk, including risk of injury and, in some cases, even extreme danger or death. The author and publisher advise readers to take full responsibility for their own safety, and truly understand and know their own limits. Before practicing the tips and sharing the knowledge described in this book, be sure that you are not taking risks beyond your level of experience, aptitude, training, and comfort level. While we do believe that reaching outside your comfort zone offers opportunities to grow, it is strongly recommended that you consult a medical and mental health professional as you start to dig deeper. Think wisely and exercise good judgment before helping others.

CONTENTS

Acknowledgments xi

Author's Note xiii

Foreword by Ben Biddick xvii

Preface xix

Part I:

An Introduction to Mental Health 1

Chapter 1: What Affects Our Mental Health? 3

Chapter 2: What is a Mental Health Emergency? 7

Chapter 3: How to Prepare Yourself as a First Responder 13

Chapter 4: Supporting Others in a Mental Health Emergency 25

Chapter 5: How to Use this Book 29

Part II:

Mental Health Conditions: The Quick Reference Guide 33

Chapter 6: Anxiety 35

Chapter 7: Depression 45

Chapter 8: Somatic Symptoms 51

Chapter 9: Personality Disorders 53

Chapter 10: Obsessive-Compulsive Behaviors 59

Chapter 11: Substance Use Disorders · 63

Chapter 12: Psychosis · 73

Chapter 13: Suicidal Behaviors · 87

Chapter 14: Trauma & Stress Related Disorders · 91

Chapter 15: Self-Injury · 99

Chapter 16: Eating Disorders · 101

Part III:

Getting Ahead of a Mental Health Crisis · 105

Chapter 17: Determining a Person's Needs · 107

Chapter 18: Support · 111

Chapter 19: How to Handle Vulnerability and
Build Mental Health Resiliency · 115

Chapter 20: De-Escalating a Situation · 119

Chapter 21: Mental Health Self-Care · 125

Conclusion: 139

Resources · 143

About the Authors · 151

Glossary of Terms · 153

Selected Bibliography · 161

DUTY TO ACT AND LEGAL CONSIDERATIONS

N SOME CASES, first responders find themselves paralyzed by the fear of lawsuits brought on by recipients of care involving consent, tort (wrongful act or an infringement of right), negligence, duty to act, and breach of duty. However, in most (if not all) cases, the first responder is protected from any legal liability for negligence, provided you do your job to the best of your ability and in accordance with the professional training you receive as a first responder. Most states have Good Samaritan laws that protect citizens, including yourself, who act independently of their "on duty" status and who provide basic voluntary emergency assistance. Please note that this law does not protect you against extreme carelessness or gross negligence.

DOCUMENTATION

As a first responder, documentation is paramount. If the encounter is not documented, then by court standards it never happened, and it is quite difficult to go off your memory to recall specific details about said event. Your profession should already require you to carry this out; for those of you acting alone, it's a good idea to get in the habit of documenting your encounters. Most first responders have standard departmental operating procedures on how to properly document encounters with subjects. These documented encounters usually include some form of SOAP (Subjective, Objective, Assessment, and Plan) notes. SOAP notes are the framework for most medical and mental health professionals and are integral for their documentation process.

ACKNOWLEDGEMENTS

THIS BOOK IS dedicated to Ms. Sumuer Watkins, for introducing us to various Mental Health training and supporting us all along the way.

Anything that you find in this book that helps in your understanding of mental health and the basic mental health emergency principles can and should be attributed to the people listed below. We are honored to have had the opportunity to work closely with most of them, as they continue to press on and improve the quality of services in the mental health community.

The mental health groups and professionals are listed here alphabetically by last name:

Groups

American Psychiatric Association
EASA | Early Assessment Support Alliance
GOBHI Greater Oregon Behavioral Health, Inc.
Maryland Department of Health and Mental Hygiene
Mayo Clinic
Missouri Department of Mental Health
NAMI | National Alliance on Mental Health
National Council for Community Behavioral Healthcare
The National Child Traumatic Stress Network
San Antonio, TX PD

Mental Health Professionals

Denise Babawale

Michelle Baldwin

Lois Bandeen

Bobbie Barbour, MA

Deidre Berens, MS, PMHNP

Lisa Bergerson

Roger Bighill

Riley Bogh

Michele Brandsma, MS,
    CADC III

Elaine Bruce

Kevin Campbell

Sarah Carpenter

Amanda Chaloux, MBA

Peggy Coreson

Rene Crump

Corin Cunningham

Clarissa Danielson

Aurora Ferreira

Elizabeth Friedman, MA

April Fresh

Lois Gilmore

Mary Graybeal

David Hamm

Frank Hanna-Williams,
    LCSW

Adelita Hinton

Roger Hayes, CADC I

Todd Jacobson, LCSW, CHC

Dawn Malcolm

Steven Manesis

Cheryl Martin

Roland Migchielsen, MS

Debbie Morrow

Ben Paz, LPC

Bud Perschek, LPC

Gayle Peterson

Marna Petersen, LPC

Jim Saxon

Dena Sites, MSW

Heike Sommer, RN, MN

Michael Walker

Martina Warnke, LPC

Andy Wasif

Jim Saxon

Kim Shillinger

Wendy Liu Skarra, MS
    LMFT

Kris Smith, CMHC

Christie Taylor, MSW

Tim Timmons, CCEP, CHP,
    CHSS

Scott Watson

AUTHOR'S NOTE
MENTAL HEALTH EMERGENCIES IN ACTION

WHEN I SET out to write this book, I simply wanted to summarize my experiences in the field of mental health, while capturing the feedback I'd received from students, colleagues, and mental health clients I have worked with. The idea was to condense all the great work from the experts, whittling it down into a convenient format that could almost fit in your pocket. But I wanted to make this more than just a book. I wanted to create a utility tool for discussion, a guidebook for breaking down barriers and overcoming social stigmas, while helping to create a movement centered on mental health as it stands today—a genuine issue of civil rights and diversity.

The day I first started jotting down the notes that would one day become the book you hold in your hands was a sunny one, a rarity in the Pacific Northwest. Our public mental health agency is located in Oregon, where (on average) our annual rainfall tends to drown out what little sunshine we see. On the off chance that you *do* get a sunny day, you tend to make it count by getting outside and enjoying it. And there were plenty of people around to enjoy it that day; more than 30,000 people had flocked to our small rural town to celebrate the thirtieth anniversary of *The Goonies*, a massive influx of people that had nearly tripled the population. The "goons" had all come to partake in the festivities, hoping to get a glimpse of their favorite childhood actors and hang out on the porch of the Goonies' house.

It was at some point in the afternoon that I received a phone call from the local law enforcement.

"Hey," said the officer, "I have one of your 'mentals' sitting in the middle of the road."

"What, you mean one of our clients?" I exclaimed. "Is everything okay?"

"No," he responded. "She's sitting in the middle of the road and won't move. All my guys are tied up on this call, and we've got a ton of people in town for the *Goonies* weekend!"

I told him that I'd be right down, and without even thinking about it, I jumped in my car and sped down the road. En route, though, a few thoughts occurred to me: "Why am I dispatching myself?" "Aren't there any other mental health professionals available that could do outreach?" But I knew it was no good; our crisis team, case managers and clinicians were all tied up. As I approached the neighborhood where our client was obstructing traffic, I quickly texted my colleague Christie Taylor, herself a clinician and case manager, to meet up with me as soon as she could. She knew this client well, and was familiar with her unique triggers.

Upon my arrival, the client was sitting in the middle of road, legs crossed, adorned in a nightgown and not much else. Law enforcement had the street cordoned off with their vehicles. I didn't really have much of a plan; keeping the client safe and getting her out of the road were my main concerns. So I walked over and simply asked her, "What's going on?"

And then, I just listened.

That day taught me three important things about mental health emergencies. First, that the need to eliminate stigma is real, and important. Second, that *anyone* can aid and assist in a crisis. And third, that the tactics used in mental health emergencies really *work*. The client was able to get up out of the street safely that day. I had conducted a swift response without even realizing it, providing much needed support while waiting for professional crisis support to arrive, who could assist her further and provide the appropriate support and services. There was virtually no difference between what I did while awaiting the arrival of professional support and someone performing rescue breathing or CPR while waiting for an ambulance.

—Nick Benas
    Astoria, Oregon 2016

FOREWORD

by Ben Biddick

THERE ARE MEN and women in every community who answer the call to public service and make it their profession to respond to emergencies. These First Responders put aside their own comfort and head out, no questions asked, whenever they're called. No matter what the emergency is or where, they move toward it in hopes of contributing their skills, resources, and training to bring resolution to whatever has gone wrong. They speed toward crime scenes, overdoses, car crashes, suicide attempts, fires, and medical emergencies without hesitation, all in hopes of saving lives and property. This is all the more impressive given that, when First Responders arrive on the scene of an emergency, they often have very little information about what has occurred; it is up to them to develop an understanding of the nature of the emergency and formulate a plan that best resolves it.

Since one in four Americans experiences a mental health issue annually (National Institute of Mental Health, 2015), First Responders—those who demand excellence of themselves and their organizations—commit to understanding the reality of mental illness as it affects the people they serve. An excellent way to do this is by reading this book.

The benefits of developing mental health literacy are innumerable. Crisis Negotiators gain the improved ability to identify whether a barricaded subject is experiencing a mental health crisis and create appropriate intervention strategies that increase the likelihood of successful de-escalation. Paramedics, Emergency Medical Technicians, and Law Enforcement Officers may find themselves able to establish rapport more effectively with those they are called on to serve, thus reducing animosity, chaos, and confrontation. Emergency medical staff may be more able to accurately assess a patient's needs and determine appropriate deployment of support services.

But by reading *Mental Health Emergencies*, first responders gain more than simply the improved ability to do their jobs. They may experience an increase in awareness, one that empowers them to get help when they need it as they attempt to cope with the chronic and traumatic stress that often accompanies a career of responding to emergencies. They may also recognize critical aspects in their interactions with coworkers, family, and friends, signs of hidden issues that have gone unnoticed for far too long. They may become more effective in encouraging and supporting their very own mental health.

After personally serving as a combat medic in the United States Army during the Global War on Terror, a combat-support military policeman, a nurse in multiple correctional institutions, a crisis negotiator, and a police officer investigating human trafficking, domestic violence, and gang-related crimes, I applaud Nick Benas, Michele Hart, and those who take the time to read their book in order to more effectively serve the public and each other. The most noble, heroic, and selfless men and women I have ever met know just how important it is to give and get help when it's needed. May the world we create every day be one where no one suffers in silence, especially our very own. To study this book is to truly invest in leaving no one behind.

—Ben Biddick, Hostage Negotiator, Janesville Police Department, Janesville Wisconsin and co-author of *Get Up: The Art of Perseverance*

PREFACE

MORE THAN 2,000 years ago, the Roman emperor Marcus Aurelius wrote, "Everything we hear is an opinion, not a fact…everything we see is a perspective, not the truth…the happiness of your life depends upon the quality of your thoughts." The stoic wisdom in these words is something I often return to; its simplicity helps get me into a truly tranquil state of mind. These thoughts and others like it are gathered together in his *Meditations*, a joyous collection of writings that can offer a framework and hope for many.

Many, but not all; for those struggling with mental health concerns or emergencies, we need more than old quotes and self-help gurus to get us through our days. (That said, reading words of inspiration and stories of happiness *are* a great start for those who are looking to employ self-care strategies in their daily lives; for those who don't, I strongly encourage you to give it a try!)

Despite how common mental health problems are, many of us make no effort to improve our situation or the situations of others. It's no surprise; we are creatures of habit, after all. We often ignore the emotional messages our body sends that tell us something is wrong. We try toughing it out like a big boy or big girl because we don't want to appear weak. Sometimes we busy ourselves with distractions; oftentimes, these take the form of self-medicating with alcohol, drugs, and other destructive behaviors. We bury our thoughts, feelings and emotions on the inside, in hopes that others won't notice. Yet the sad truth is that these things will always affect those around us. The anxiety, depression and other symptoms we experience *do* impact others.

Part I

An Introduction to Mental Health

Wнат is a mental health crisis or mental health emergency? A mental health crisis or emergency, in its simplest form, is when your brain and body are out of step with each other. It is an unstable moment of time where a person's emotional control is disrupted by unusual and critical changes.

These changes are introduced by forms of stress and changes in one's environment. For every individual, there is a different trigger that affects the person. Even the healthiest individuals experience mental health crises, and it is even more normal when there's a response to abnormal events, especially those which involve trauma and physical injury. In these cases, it is the first responder who is best equipped to decipher certain stresses and assess the necessary care.

The following material is well-suited for early adopters that are new to the emergency profession, seasoned veterans and even concerned citizens. The content is easily digestible, distilled down from lengthy technical jargon to provide a basic understanding of the different mental health conditions and diagnosable illnesses that many are suffering with. The book is simple to use and is a good resource to quickly navigate back to when you want to clarify certain terms and tactics. It will walk you through all the steps and help you develop "muscle memory" and quick recall for when you go on to do more comprehensive study and training in the mental health crisis arena.

CHAPTER 1

What Affects Our Mental Health?

A PERSON'S MENTAL AND emotional health is shaped by their many life experiences, especially those in early childhood. Genetic and biological factors also play a role, but even these can be shaped and molded by one's experiences. Experiences that have been noted as influencing one's mental health condition include:

- **Poor connection or attachment to your primary care-taker/parent/guardian early in life.** Feeling lonely, isolated, unsafe, confused, or abused verbally, physically or sexually as an infant or young child can lead to an inability to form lasting personal connections and may promote a tendency to self-isolate, which increases one's risk for a variety of mental health disorders.

- **Traumas or serious losses, especially early on in life.** The death of a parent or other traumatic experiences, such as a car accident, being involved in a natural disaster, serving in a combat zone, or prolonged hospitalization can affect your likelihood of falling prey to a mental illness and experiencing symptoms like anxiety and depression, which can worsen over time.

- **Learned helplessness.** Negative experiences that lead to a belief that you're helpless, and that you have little control over the situations in your life, can result in feelings of anxiety and depression.

- **Illness.** Physical illness and ailments, especially when chronic, disabling, or isolating, can negatively impact your mental health.

- **Side effects of medications.** Unwanted side effects from prescription medications (especially in older people, who may be taking a variety of medications) can cause imbalances in brain and body chemistry, leading to or exacerbating one's mental illness.

- **Substance abuse.** Alcohol and drug abuse can both cause mental health problems and make preexisting mental or emotional problems worse.

Thankfully, regardless of whatever factors have shaped your mental and emotional health, it's never too late to make changes that will counteract any risk factors and improve your psychological well-being.

A BRIEF HISTORY OF MENTAL HEALTH

1.0 ERA: Prior to the 1960s, many people suffering with mental health illness were treated in secure facilities, such as state hospitals, for a host of reasons. Of course, having long term psychiatric facilities for people with mental disorders is a practice that goes way back in time. The Germans had a building built specifically to house mentally ill people dating back to 1784, named Vienna's Narrenturm, which in German means "fools tower." (Rout, S., *Vienna Direct*, 2017)

2.0 ERA: With the deinstitutionalizations of state hospitals in the late 1960s and early 1970s came the onset of a new socio-political environment. New psychotropic medications were arriving on the scene to treat different disorders, while a shift to Social Security Income (SSI) and Social Security Disability (SSD) now provided those in need with more support mechanisms. Yet still, many individuals ended up on the street because there were not enough resources to address their needs.

3.0 ERA: Federally funded, community based mental health programs began to sprout up in the 1980s to early 2000s, alongside a renewed criminalization of the mentally ill. Common misconceptions, encouraged by the media and perpetuated in Hollywood, led to the public belief that the mentally ill are dangerous and that their actions are unpredictable. And, because first responders and law enforcement weren't properly trained to handle the new strain—they didn't know how to handle the individuals' suffering—many ended up in jail or emergency rooms for prolonged stays without proper care. Because of the existing tactics in place and lack of mental health resources involving first responders, there have even been reported instances of individuals becoming aggravated and escalated to levels of aggression that, in some cases, could have been prevented.

4.0 ERA: Moving forward to the present day, fully integrated mobile mental health units are starting to pop up. Mental health professionals, trained first responders, and social workers integrated with law enforcement, firefighting, EMT units, and our public-school systems are now in a position to provide the proper care to those who need it. You—the first responder on the front lines—are being called on to address mental health concerns and crises in your community, to the best of your ability.

CHAPTER 2

What is a Mental Health Emergency?

MENTAL ILLNESSES AFFECT one's ability to think, feel and relate to others. The more serious kinds of illness cause people to live in an altered state which, no matter how unreal it may seem to the outside observer, is all too real for the one experiencing it. Some mental illness is severe enough that anyone can recognize and label it; others manifest in more subtle ways that blur the lines between what is considered normal and abnormal. When these factors interfere with daily living and escalate to crisis levels, they often result in a mental health emergency.

The following may be factors in a mental health emergency and will need the intervention of a mental health professional after the crisis or mental health emergency is resolved:

- Inability to sleep, restlessness
- Feeling "blue," hopeless, or helpless most of the time

- Concentration problems that impede basic thinking and ability to recall, or interfere with relationships, work or home life
- Using food, drugs, or alcohol to cope with difficult emotions
- Negative or self-destructive thoughts or fears that you can't control
- Thoughts of harming oneself, including suicide and death

> If you or anyone you know is experiencing a mental health emergency and is in need of immediate support and attention, call the National Suicide Prevention Line at **1-800-273-8255.** Trained crisis workers are available to help, 24 hours a day.

If these conditions often develop early and only worsen over time, why do they result in mental health crises? Why do individuals not seek treatment for their long-term mental illnesses? The truth is that mental health and mental illness has taken a back seat in healthcare for years. People are unfairly blamed for behaviors which are simply symptoms of their mental health conditions. To this day, we see discrimination against those with mental illness as their fight for civil rights continues. All too often, these stigmas regarding mental health are based solely on fear and a lack of proper understanding. If you or a loved one has ever experienced this discrimination, you can appreciate the true importance of this book.

As a first responder, you can be instrumental in disseminating this information amongst your ranks. Change *can* start with you. In 1979, a group of concerned family members and friends of the mentally ill formed National Alliance for the Mentally Ill (NAMI), an organization to help reduce the stigma of mental illness. NAMI remains the nation's largest grassroots organization, and is staffed by volunteers working to help improve the lives of those with mental illness.

Their work has never been more important, as the number of Americans affected by mental illness continues to grow. According to studies performed by medical experts, roughly one in four individuals seeking medical help for their physical concerns usually has an undetected mental illness/disorder adding to or compounding their situation. These issues start surfacing in late teens/early adulthood, yet people continue to become ill without seeking help from a mental health professional. Why?

It's not for lack of available resources; many medical doctors have extensive backgrounds in mental health, and can identify signs and symptoms of mental illness in their patients. With the new advancements in health care, patients even have the option to see a mental health professional right there in the doctor's office.

So why are most people reluctant to address their mental health needs? There are many reasons; here are a few that you may come across when you encounter the public:

- **Some people mistakenly see mental health problems as something you should "walk off."** For example, one generalization is that men are more inclined to keep their feelings to themselves.

- **Many people think that if they do seek help, the treatment will be expensive, or carry risk of side effects.**

The belief that the only treatment options available are medication (which comes with unwanted side effects) or therapy (which can be lengthy, difficult to navigate and expensive), often serves as a roadblock for those seeking help with their mental illness. The truth is that whatever your issues, there are a multitude of services and support networks available, as well as self-care information like hobbies such as hunting or hiking, and physical exercises like running, lifting, martial arts classes, and yoga to help you improve the way you feel and experience greater mental and emotional well-being.

- **They may not view their illness as legitimate, or warranting concern.** In some societies and certain conservative religious sects, mental and emotional issues are less legitimate than physical health issues. They're seen as a sign of weakness or a result of one's own actions. In some countries and communities, mental illness is looked at as the result of "witchcraft" or "voodoo;" in other words, they don't see the point in treating the patient for what is perceived as an external issue.

- **They may think their feelings are natural—even expected—based on circumstance.** The issue may be viewed as simply a natural part of a larger experience, such as grief or loss. Loss is painful, and grief over loss is a natural part of life. There is no right or wrong way to grieve, but there *are* healthy ways to cope with the pain and express your emotions in ways that allow you to heal. While many people can manage their emotions, the truth is that some emotions can be threatening. We can become overwhelmed by threats and stresses in our lives and lose the ability to keep things in balance. When this happens, our alarm system goes off, and we go into a "fight, flight, or freeze" mode and lose control of our behavior. Freeze indicates a person's inability to manage the situation at hand, resulting in a complete shutdown.

The following signs and symptoms may be present when you encounter someone experiencing a mental health emergency:

- **Mood Swings**: Big shifts in emotions that are rapid in nature.

- **Social Withdrawal**: The person is isolating and withdrawing interest in others, including friends and family.

- **Disorientation**: The person is having problems with their thinking, their basic recall/memory, speech, and concentration. They may be having a difficult time trying to focus and process what you are asking of them.

- **Overstimulated**: The person shows sensitivity to light, sights, sounds, crowds, touches and smells, and they avoid anything that is overstimulating. They are also overwhelmed by the accident scene or area of natural disaster.

- **Apathy**: The person has a loss of desire to participate in any activity or follow your directions.

- **Disconnection**: The person has a sense of un-reality and feels disconnected from themselves or their surroundings. If psychosis is present, they may be seeing things or hearing things that are not there, but which are real to them.

- **Illogical Thought**: Unusual or exaggerated beliefs about personal powers to understand meanings or influence events, illogical or regressive thinking (returning to earlier states of mind).

- **Nervousness**: Fear or suspiciousness of others or a strong feeling of anxiety towards the unknown.

- **Unusual Behavior**: When the person acts peculiar, odd or uncharacteristic of themselves.

- **Appetite Changes**: Eating too much or too little.

- **Sleep Hygiene**: Sleeplessness or too much sleep.

CHAPTER 3

How to Prepare Yourself as a First Responder

ENTAL HEALTH "ISSUES," "concerns," "crises" and "emergencies" affect us all in one way or another. As a first responder, your job is a difficult one. Mental health can complicate things, turning basic routine calls into bigger, more demanding emergencies. Emotion and chaos adds another layer to your routine and creates difficulty when assessing the individual on the scene. As a first responder, you are equipped with some of the best training in the world. You are likely very comfortable addressing safety issues, physical ailments and physical injuries of the subjects at the scene.

But the presence of mental health crises and co-morbidity (meaning the mental health issues are co-occurring with substance use disorders) complicates matters quite a bit. These situations can be overwhelming, on top of your existing level of stress from needing to specialize in these difficult areas. You need to be able to decipher between the stress of the critical incident at hand and a mental health emergency. Even though mental health is confusing, unseen, and difficult to triage at first, the more you are exposed to it, the more you will start to become comfortable with handling these concerns.

That said, it is important to understand that even as you start to grow and gain confidence, you must not become complacent. In the situations you are presented with, there are no scripts, and you must do the best with the resources you are equipped with, while still relying heavily on the aid and support of medical and mental health professionals when necessary.

After you size up the scene, make sure you, your staff and the people on the scene are safe. Safety is paramount. When you arrive on scene, you are expected to gather quick specifics of the situation, i.e. survey the scene for hazards, determine the mechanism(s) of physical injury if they are present, isolate bodily substances, grab a quick tally of the individuals, assess for possible threats, and then assess the needs of the situation, the person in crisis and quickly build rapport so you may gain a grasp on the situation.

Sounds easy, right? Nope. You are the front line. You are the help and the one to assist. Whether you are a police officer, firefighter, EMT, paramedic, military service member, federal agent, correctional officer, life guard, school teacher or pastor well-versed in pre-medical care for medical emergencies, you will be looked upon to provide exactly the right kind of support in the absence of trained mental health professional when the need arises.

The first responder should develop an ability to recognize, treat (in the most rudimentary way), and help prevent escalation of other crises when it applies to mental health. It is important to note that this guide will not prepare you for the treatment and diagnosis of individuals; let's leave that up to the professionals. The information provided is to help you become more comfortable with the prevalence of mental health disorders and the issues and concerns that present themselves every day.

To summarize, the first responder must:

- Stay calm and impassive (mask your feelings) in their approach

- Be aware of the safety risks: weapons, and any physical hazards like broken glass, sharp objects, water, gas, fire, and tall structures

- Build rapport quickly and continue to maintain that trust

- Give swift, early treatment

- Call appropriate help and/or emergency services or the medical oversight embedded in your teams

- Remember their own needs as a first responder

EMERGENCY SUPPORT VS. PROFESSIONAL SUPPORT

You *are* a professional, and the continuum of care usually starts with you, but long term care needs to be entrusted to the mental health professionals and the individuals advocating for their care. Unfortunately, there is no one quick fix for mental health or substance use disorders, but having you on the front lines with a clear understanding of these concerns helps the safety and well-being of others, and contributes to the whole continuum of care.

You are encouraged to seek additional training and appropriate professional guidance from local agencies in your area. For those feeling more ambitious, we would recommend taking the time to become a mental health guru and look to model agencies who are already equipped with Counselors in Training (CIT) and active groups where mental health professionals are accompanying first responders on emergency calls. In the coming years, mental health emergency training will become more commonplace, just like physical medical response, first aid, and CPR. It won't be unusual to see employers adopting a mental health emergency training as a requirement.

Personal Aims and Objectives

The first responder should consider the following priorities in the performance of their duty:

- Be aware of your own needs as a first responder and the objectives, outcomes and protocol(s) of your job

- Understand your own comfort zone, abilities, weaknesses and limitations, as well as strengths

- Learn how to really listen and exercise empathy

- Stay calm in your approach and be clear and concise with your communication and economy of body language

- Stay safe always

ADDRESSING DIVERSITY IN MENTAL HEALTH EMERGENCIES

As a first responder, you will have loved ones, colleagues, friends, and family who are affected by mental health concerns. At the same time, be aware that you will encounter a very diverse population of people in your daily life, many of whom have their own unique set of personal issues. Understand that your attitudes, feelings and beliefs are not the lens that others may look through. Along with the common signs and symptoms of mental health issues, individuals may be suffering in silence or handling crisis differently because of their certain set of circumstances, which may not be easily seen when you make your contact. A major tenet of *Mental Health Emergencies* is straight-up empathy and listening. It is important for you as a first responder to reassess your preconceived attitudes about people and mental health. You must avoid any premature conclusions based on what you and your colleagues, friends or family connections have experienced.

Understanding Youths in a Mental Health Emergency

Mental health literacy is very important for those who live and work with the youth. Mental health problems are very common amongst youths, and many develop during adolescence. Compounding things, youths have a very different experience when dealing with mental illness and emotional stress, and may want to exercise a different approach than adults. Young people may also not be well informed, but the sooner they receive help, the sooner they can begin to work towards a positive outcome.

Before reaching out to a youth, please consider the following:
- The role and relationship you have with the youth

- Ethical guidelines, objectives and protocols of your job as a first responder

- Legal requirements and ramifications of extending outside the scope of your current job responsibilities

- Professional restrictions in your line work

- Role of family members

- Young person's right to privacy

- Your realistic ability to help

It is important to note that the professional knowledge presented here does not equip you to supersede any mandatory legal reporting requirements, any professional policies of an organization or regulatory body, or the protocols of your agency. A friendly reminder: always consider your own safety, the safety of your team and your potential effectiveness before interacting with anyone in a mental health crisis or emergency, including individuals you don't know and are approaching for the first time. If you feel that you are not ready to handle the situation at hand, it is okay to have a colleague step in if they are equipped to continue the proper continuum of care.

Understanding the LGBTIQ Community in Mental Health Emergencies

As a first responder, it is important that you develop sensitivities and broaden your knowledge of sexuality and gender. When dealing with diverse populations, the first responder must come to understand that gender isn't a binary, male/ female system—it's a spectrum. Gender and sexuality can be very fluid, and there is a large variety of individuals who would categorize and identify themselves differently than they might appear. Just as is the case for heterosexuality/homosexuality, in which not everyone's sexual attraction is to opposite sex members, the same applies to other identities. Gender and sexuality may change over time, and a person using a LGBTIQ label may hold a variety of identities (LGBTIQ stands for "Lesbian, Gay, Bisexual, Transgender, Intersex, and Queer and (or Questioning).

Avoid using pronouns like "he" and "she" when speaking to someone during a mental health emergency. When the time is appropriate, ask them how they would like to identify or refer to them by their first name. Do not ask questions about the LGBTIQ experience or address habits or gender unless it is relevant to assisting that particular person and their current needs.

Certain religious sects and cultures also place a large stigma on the LGBTIQ community; this, combined with our already judgmental societal norms, has brought a great deal of suffering to LGBTIQ individuals. They can end up developing a lot of negative attitudes about themselves that become internalized and cause a great deal of distress and it turn many times can result in a mental health emergency.

If a person is experiencing mental health problems due to bullying, harassment or discrimination related to their LGBTIQ experience, you as the first responder should let the person know that they can report it to the authorities and that it is safe to do so. Make sure to document the information accordingly.

Understanding Veterans and Military Personnel in Mental Health Emergencies

As a first responder, you may meet current or former members of the armed forces, who may be having a hard time readjusting to civilian life. They may seem to always be on edge, always on the verge of exploding, or appear emotionally numb and disconnected from the rest of society. These are common symptoms that today's veterans are facing, all of which are typically grouped under the umbrella term post-traumatic stress disorder (PTSD). Without the rush of being in a combat zone, veterans may describe themselves as feeling strange or even dead inside. Many veterans are drawn to things that offer the familiar adrenaline rush, whether it's caffeinated energy drinks, drugs, violent video games, driving recklessly, or daredevil and extreme sports.

When working with a veteran or member of the military dealing with mental health issues relating to their experience, remind them that healing doesn't mean forgetting what happened or those who died. What it does mean is that they need to learn to look at their role more realistically. Is the amount of responsibility they're assuming reasonable? Helping them to honestly assess their responsibility frees them to move on and grieve their losses.

Service members often feel like the civilians in their life can't understand them. They feel like other people have a hard time relating since they haven't been in the service or "seen" the things they have. But people don't have to have gone through the exact same experiences to be able to offer support. What matters is that the person you're turning to cares about you, is a good, non-judgmental listener, and is a strong source of support.

Understanding Older Adults in Mental Health Emergencies

You will need to exercise the most amount of patience while working with older adults. You may be used to working at warp speed in an accelerated environment, where your primary focus is to get the crisis or emergency resolved and rapidly respond to that next call. Older adults may complicate your job by having dementia or memory loss because of old age; this will confuse everything you've learned thus far about mental health. Do not bring attention to the fact that they are getting frustrated with your help and questions, as this will make it more difficult to build rapport with that person.

You may find yourself assisting with certain physical ailments, or helping them while they move about and get comfortable. Engage the assistance of team members or bystanders if you are helping them walk, move around in their wheelchair, climb stairs, navigate obstacles, or simply getting them to sit in a comfortable spot. Understand that "accidents" will happen, and you may be addressing missed bowel movements and bathroom calls.

When working with the elderly population, do not assume the individual has limitations or disabilities due to their age. If they are brief in their communication style, don't assume that they don't understand your questions and directions. If they seem a little confused or disorientated at first, make sure to handle the individuals consistently, the same way you handle everyone else when you approach on an emergency call. Speak slowly and repeat your questions back several times until they understand what you are sharing with them.

Exercise your patience skills, remembering to slow down your actions and communication style. Speak slowly, projecting your voice if the individual is hard of hearing, and repeat your questions, their needs and concerns back to them so they understand. If the person is overwhelmed, take some time out and revisit the communication while they reorient themselves. Never assume that the individual doesn't understand, and never speculate as to what the person is suffering from.

MENTAL HEALTH OVERSIGHT AS A FIRST RESPONDER

It is assumed that you, as a first responder, have an existing medical mental oversight and quality assurance in place as you act in the line of duty. It is also assumed that you have the proper training and protocols in place to protect the safety and quality of care for the individuals you meet.

But with some smaller outfits and agencies, you may not have that luxury. The following information will help guide you in any gray areas you may have. The information you glean from this book should help you and your team build an approach to improve the quality of care for those suffering in a mental health emergency. This overview of basic mental health knowledge for mental health concerns and/or emergencies will help you function at a much higher level in any environment or unusual circumstance.

Mental health emergency first responders shall:

- Exercise safety.
- Develop a basic understanding of the most common mental health concerns.
- Recognize and assess the seriousness of the mental health concern, crisis, or emergency the person is dealing with.

- Exercise active listening steps:

  + Restate what you heard the person say

  + Use clear, direct, person-focused language

  + Pause before responding

  + Ask for clarification if needed; never assume

  + Don't pretend to know what the person thinks before they do

  + Give micro responses: nod your head, lean in with your body and make eye contact

- Exercise empathy. Empathy is the awareness of the feelings and emotions of other people. It is the link between the self and others because it is how we, as individuals, understand what others are experiencing as if we were feeling it ourselves.

- Continue your mental health literacy and education, referring often to the quick reference guide in the back of this book. As a first responder, you should continue to work on your skills and learn as much as you can about mental health and substance use disorders so you can develop your sensitivity and build on those areas where you are qualified to offer aid.

As a first responder, you are usually entering a scene with limited medical gear and mental health capabilities. All the same, you are answering the call to help, providing care to the injured and those in distress. Your skills are expected to be polished and current, and your execution efficient.

CHAPTER 4

Supporting Others in a Mental Health Emergency

A S EXPLAINED EARLIER, there is an undisputed connection between positive social relationships and greater mental and emotional health, including lower stress, improved resilience, better mood and higher self-esteem.

Researchers are discovering that the greatest benefit of social connection stems from the act of giving to others. By measuring hormones and brain activity when people are being helpful to others, researchers have discovered that being generous triggers an immense pleasure response in the brain. Just as we're hard-wired to be social, we're also hard-wired to give to others. What this means is that you have more control over your emotional health and happiness than you may have imagined.

That said, supporting others *is* a learned skill; one that, with practice, you can develop over time. As a first responder, you have made a commitment to learning how best to care for and support others in the moment when they need it most. While for some, supporting others may not be instinctive and at first may even seem unrewarding, like any learned behavior it can be developed. Starting small, dedicating even small amounts of time and energy to helping others, will boost your efficiency and effectiveness on the job.

The landscape of today's emergency calls and run-in society means a more complex and diverse person suffering, which in turn means your job is becoming more and more difficult. A mentally healthy, well-educated first responder is vital to achieve good results, provide excellent aid, and assist the lives of those suffering in a mental health emergency. Learning how to respond appropriately to a mental health emergency and how to motivate others to act swiftly, including those suffering, can make all the difference in the world. By using the proper talking tactics, accountability, and the information provided in this guide, you create a safer and healthier space in your operations during a mental health crisis. Don't underestimate this; you may just save someone's life someday. The tips in this chapter may already be a part of your professional toolkit or agency's protocols, but use these as a friendly reminder to reset, refresh and add to your existing training regimens:

- Be very clear and concise in your approach. This includes the words you choose when communicating and the economy of your body language (overall energy, motion, telling signs and dramatics). Strengthen your message by keeping to a slow cadence, using brief phrases, and repeating when necessary. Always be confident and upbeat with the delivery of your message.

- Deliver communication as soon as possible and keep the individual(s) informed on the next action steps when necessary.

- Encourage the person to participate in the decision-making process.

- Exercise patience, tolerance, understanding and (in some cases) firm but respectful disagreement.

- Do not get into any arguments with the individual experiencing the mental health crisis. Be courteous to the person suffering; this will help you build rapport rapidly, and relieve any anxiety or insecurity that they are dealing with in the moment. It is important to be genuine in your responses and not smother the individual. If the person is in psychosis, acknowledge the images and voices they are sharing with you. Be reflexive in your responses by repeating back what they are telling you.

- Be a team player and do your part to help solve the problems of the current situation. This is another sure-fire way to build rapport quickly, showing that you are going out of your way to assist. It is important to note that you aren't just doing things directly for that person; it is a collaboration, a team effort. Finding a cause is not necessary to creating solutions.

- Use rating scales 1–10 to assess how the person feels they are coping in the moment (0 being no coping and 10 being perfect coping).

- Motivational Interviewing (MI): This is a basic communication method which incorporates a person-centered approach. There are five basic tenants to MI. :

    + Express empathy through reflective listening. Paraphrase back what the person is stating and be in the moment.

+ Develop discrepancy. Differentiate between clients' goals or values and their current behavior.

+ Avoid arguing and confrontation.

+ Adjust to client resistance rather than opposing it directly; invite new perspectives without forcing them.

+ Support self-efficacy and optimism by assisting the person with finding their strengths and helping them understand how to use them by finding other approaches.

• Reflective Communication Techniques: This involves actively listening to person. Seek to understand what the individual is saying and offer ideas back to them.

CHAPTER 5

How to Use this Book

THIS BOOK IS organized into chapters, each of which deals with one of the most common diagnosable mental health conditions. These cover everything from mild anxiety and depression to the more severe bipolar disorder, schizophrenia and self-injury behaviors. Within each section there are easy-to-understand descriptions and explanations of several kinds of mental illnesses.

Located in the back of the book is a quick guide to mental health resources that are great for providing additional information, along with a glossary of mental health terms. For those who feel that they already have a good understanding of these mental health illnesses, we recommend that you take the time to re-read the definitions, signs, and symptoms throughout. Too often, we assign definitions in our heads based on the labels that are thrown around in our everyday language. By taking the time to read everything through, you help clarify any misconceptions that you may have. The most important job of these definitions is providing an understanding of how these things can shape an individual's behavior and clear the lens that you are currently looking through.

Whether you're a brand-new officer, firefighter, medic, nurse, first responder, teacher, pastor, or just a concerned citizen who would like to be informed about how to handle a mental health emergency, you can read this book from back to front and keep it handy for moments when you get confused and need step-by-step instructions.

If you're already an experienced professional, you can treat this book as a general reference and jump into the chapters that suit your needs, using the quick reference guide and glossary in the back for rapid recall. Just remember that there is always room for growth and skill development, and when you have a question or need a little assistance when working with your team, this is a great place to turn.

CONDITIONS, LABELS, DIAGNOSES AND INJURIES

Conditions, labels, diagnoses and descriptions of injuries are present throughout this book. These include the signs (things people see) and the symptoms (things people feel) of mental health issues. Please note that not all mental illnesses/disorders are covered in this book. Please refer to the DSM-5 (Diagnostic and Statistical Manual of Mental Disorders, 2013) if you're curious about an illness or disorder that we didn't include. Just keep in mind that the DSM-5 is a manual intended to be used by professionals. Using it may make you feel uncomfortable at times; it is sometimes too easy to identify with some passages and begin to worry that you have every disorder under the sun.

Our advice is that it's healthier not to borrow worry, so it might be better to find your light reading elsewhere.

PART II

Mental Health Conditions:

The Quick Reference Guide

THE FOLLOWING PAGES will be your guide to providing much-needed care and support to the people who are in distress and who most need your help. *Mental Health Emergencies* is a comprehensive guide to mental and emotional health crises and concerns, providing overviews of the most common mental health problems, as well as expert guidance on more serious problems, including self-injury, eating disorders, substance abuse, psychosis, and suicidal thoughts.

The content that follows was developed from the best-practices of psychiatry, psychology, mental health case management and counseling. You must continue to operate within the scope of your job description and have a clear understanding that the information provided in this guidebook will not place you in the position to be a licensed or certified mental health professional. By no means should you feel qualified to be diagnosing mental illness or prescribing medications. We ask that you exercise good common sense and professional judgment. In certain professions, as a first responder, you have the luxury of leaning on the authority of a medical or clinical supervisor. In those fields where you don't have that luxury, please rely on outside mental health professionals for professional support.

CHAPTER 6

Anxiety

DEFINING ANXIETY

Anxiety is common. For most of us, it is a normal response mechanism to the stress in our daily lives. Anxiety is the body's alarm system which helps us pay attention when it is necessary and can alert us to certain situations, including extreme dangers. It's a useful tool, built-in during human evolution, but can be a burden now that we don't have to fight off lions, tigers and other natural predators. There are many causes of anxiety that are unknown, but many suspect factors which include psychological (emotional state of the person), environmental (home environments, school, work and social settings) and genetic.

When we say anxiety is common, we mean that everyone experiences it, including you. When we say that someone is anxious, we simply mean that they are uneasy, or always nervous, worried about an unforeseen event or uncertain about future events.

Some manage their anxiety levels better than others. For some, anxiety can be very debilitating. Per the National Alliance of Mental Health (NAMI), it is estimated that approximately 18 percent of the U.S. population suffers from an anxiety disorder. That number is quite substantial; it also means the people around you in your day-to-day life are impacted severely by their anxiety symptoms. They have difficulty going about their daily activities and suffer disruptions to the "normal," things most people take for granted. If anxiety symptoms go untreated, there is an increased likelihood of the individual experiencing a mental health crisis or emergency.

When anxiety starts to become a burden, manifesting as extreme anxiousness, excessive fear and worry, it starts impacting the individual and becomes a mental health disorder or illness.

Anxiety disorders are very common, and many individuals are affected by one at some time in their life. Thankfully, there are treatments for these anxiety disorders, and if these disorders are managed properly, there should be no real concerns. It is only when these disorders are ignored or mismanaged that they can exacerbate other problem areas of one's health.

WHAT DOES ANXIETY LOOK LIKE IN A MENTAL HEALTH EMERGENCY?

Physical indicators of anxiety include:

- Rapid heart beats

- Shortness of breath and trouble breathing comfortably

- Fatigue that sets in

- The individual shares with you that they are having insomnia

- Upset stomach

- Frequent bowel movements and urination

- Profuse sweating

- Twitching and tremors in the body

- Muscle tension

- Shortness of breath

Mental and emotional indicators of anxiety include:

- Fear of the unknown (the individual may share concerns on future events)

- Excessive worry

- Fear of losing control or going crazy

- Parenthesis (numbing or tingling sensations)

- Fear of dying

- They tell you they feel a "doom" and "dread" feeling

- Tension, agitation, restlessness and feeling "cagey," a feeling of cautiousness

- Anticipating worst case scenarios and negative outcomes

TYPES OF ANXIETY DISORDERS

Anxiety disorders vary in their signs and symptoms and may require different types of self-help, support and treatments. The DSM-5 (Diagnostic Service Manual) outlines the following anxiety disorders:

Generalized Anxiety Disorder (GAD)

Generalized anxiety disorder (GAD) is chronic and exaggerated worrying about everyday life. The person suffering with GAD will experience a variety of symptoms which will include headaches, tension, nausea, and exhaustion (due to their other symptoms) that takes hold and makes it very difficult for that person to carry out their daily activities. This excessive worry can consume hours of one's day, making it extremely difficult for them to focus.

Panic Disorder

A panic disorder is categorized as the frequent, routine experience of panic attacks. A panic attack is defined as a sudden and overwhelming feeling of terror that usually appears without warning and will repeat itself. It comes about unexpectedly, and may peak within 10 minutes of the episode's start. When in mid-panic attack, many of the following symptoms are present:

- Sweating

- Shaking and body tremors

- Shortness of breath, pounding heart, palpitations and a rapid heart rate

- Sensations of smothering or choking

- Chest pains

- Discomfort

- Nausea, abdominal distress

- Dizziness, feeling faint or unsteady

- Feelings of unreality or being detached from oneself

- Fears of losing control or going "crazy"
- Fear of death
- Feeling numbness or tingling
- Hot flashes or chills

Panic disorders can resemble heart conditions and it very common for people to mistake it as a heart attack. A person suffering a panic attack will experience chest pain, heart palpitations, dizziness, upset stomach and shortness of breath. Typically, more than one in five people will experience at least one panic attack in their lifetime, but few will go on to develop other panic disorders.

Phobias

Phobia describes anxiety disorders that are based around an irrational fear. "Fear" is defined as an emotional response from a perceived threat and the fear of the unknown. The nature of the irrational fear can vary; for example, agoraphobia is the fear of being in a situation where one is around a lot of people, where escaping may be difficult or embarrassing to the individual.

This fear is typically out of proportion to the actual situation and generally lasts six months or more, causing problems in daily functioning.

Social Anxiety Disorder

When a person has a persistent fear of one or more social or performance situations in which the person is exposed to unfamiliar people or to perceived scrutiny by others, they are understood to be suffering from social anxiety disorder.

Separation Anxiety Disorder

Separation anxiety disorder describes a situation in which a person is extremely fearful or anxious about separation from those whom the individual is attached to. The feeling is beyond appropriate for the person's age, persists at least four weeks in children and six months in adults, and causes problems in functioning.

ANXIETY AND FINANCIAL ISSUES

It should come as no surprise that mental health problems and financial difficulties often go hand in hand. Of all the things that people experience anxiety over, money is perhaps the most common. It is important to note that having mental health problems does *not* indicate the inability to manage money; we can all relate to the stresses that surround money. However, mental health problems can often *contribute* to financial difficulties, and those financial difficulties may in turn contribute to one's mental health, anxiousness and depression, creating a vicious cycle.

Specific sources of financial difficulties for people with mental health problems may include the following:

- Debt incurred to support a drug, alcohol, or gambling problem

- Increased medical expenses (which can become a continuous cycle if they have poor physical and mental health)

- Overspending when in a manic or depressed state

- Job instability or unemployment associated with episodic mental illness

---

TREATING ANXIETY

You may note that anxiety is one of the most common mental health concerns you will see during an emergency encounter. You may even start noticing changes within yourself as you respond to high stress situations and traumatic events like fires, car accidents and natural catastrophes.

It is recommended that a person experiencing anxiousness and anxiety-like symptoms consult and work with a mental health professional. While working with a professional, a care plan is devised that can address the specific needs of that individual. A good plan would be driven by the consumer receiving the mental health services and not driven by the mental health professional. A good care plan would also likely include some therapeutic strategies, meditation, stress-management techniques, group therapy work, medication management (in specific cases), as well as self-care, anti-stressing "life hacks" to be carried out at home in the person's daily life.

It is a good idea to become familiar with the following concepts of professional mental health treatment, as they may surface in your conversations with people out in the community and/or with team members involved in the emergency call you are responding to.

Cognitive Behavioral Therapy (CBT)

Cognitive behavioral therapy comprises of individual talk therapy that is focused on behavioral changes and increased awareness of the individual's behaviors and thinking. The therapy has a very short term focus with the approach of accelerating the individual's emotional recovery.

Eye Movement Desensitization and Reprocessing (EMDR)

Eye Movement Desensitization and Reprocessing (EMDR) is a new and progressive therapeutic model that includes the use of proprietary bilateral stimulation/eye movement. Developed by Francine Shapiro in 1987, the technique focuses on healing individuals from emotional distress, usually caused by traumatic life events. A Kaiser Permanete study has shown very high success rates with single-trauma and multi-trauma victims suffering with symptoms of Post-Traumatic Stress Disorder (PTSD) and anxiety symptoms. The individuals' diagnoses went away after several sessions with a professional. For more information, check out the EMDR Institute, Inc. in the Resources section of this book.

Dialectical Behavioral Therapy (DBT)

Dialectical behavioral therapy is a therapy designed to help people suffering from mood disorders, as well as those who need to change patterns of behavior that are not helpful, such as self-harm, suicidal ideation, and substance abuse. This approach works towards helping people increase their emotional and cognitive regulation by learning about the triggers that lead to reactive states and helping to assess which coping skills to apply to help avoid undesired reactions. DBT assumes that people are doing their best but lack the skills needed to succeed, or who are influenced by positive reinforcement or negative reinforcement that interferes with their ability to function appropriately.

DBT is a modified form of cognitive behavioral therapy. There are four key skills in DBT: Distress Tolerance, to assist a person to cope better with painful events; Mindfulness, which helps a person more fully experience a moment and provide tools to overcome habitual and negative judgments about self and others; Emotional Regulation, which helps a person to recognize more clearly what they feel and not be overwhelmed by it; and Interpersonal Effectiveness, which provides the person with new tools to express beliefs, needs, set limits and negotiate solutions to problems.

Group Therapy

Group therapy provides a way to access the behaviors, interactions, and awareness of individuals suffering with anxiousness and anxiety-like signs and symptoms. The group dynamic is known to bring about encouragement, hope, information, knowledge, interpersonal teaching, learning and wisdom from individuals who have been there before. Having peers present provides a supportive atmosphere for others in the group and allows room for exceptional gratitude and wellness. The group dynamic also allows for individuals to practice positive behavioral patterns in a group setting.

SELF-HELP HACKS AND COPING MECHANISMS FOR ANXIETY

- Visualize what you want the end of your anxiety to look like, define the steps needed to reach that state, and work toward that goal.

- Yoga works on the mind and body connection and is meditative by nature.

- Mindfulness and meditation provide a great source for stress relief. You can find plenty of resources in books and classes, both online and offline.

- Implementing morning rituals and priming, such as deep breathing and visualization of the people and experiences you are grateful for in life can center you for the day ahead.

- Avoid caffeinated beverages such as soda, energy drinks, tea and coffee. Caffeine is a culprit known to induce and worsen an individual's anxiety symptoms.

- Martial arts, Brazilian Jiu-Jitsu (for the more serious) or Tai Chi and Kung Fu (for lower impact) lets you move your body in a focused way.

- Pursue hobbies and mindfulness activities that include focus, such as painting, pottery, archery, marksmanship, hunting and recreational activities that keep your mind and body occupied.

CHAPTER 7

Depression

THE DSM-5 DEFINES depression thusly: "Depression is a very common and serious mental illness that negatively affects how you feel, the way you think, and how you act." People lose interest in the things they enjoy and withdraw from the relationships they once engaged in. Note that depression is not a specific disorder in the DSM-5. It is categorized under Depressive Disorders, which are described according to duration, timing, and presumed etiology. Depression is a blanket term, commonly used to refer to a number of interrelated symptoms.

Nevertheless, depression is considered to be a very serious mental health condition, one which can be moderate to severe in its symptoms. It is a pervasive illness that can lead to certain disruptions in a person's life due to persistent feelings of sadness and guilt.

Depression is an experience all too common for many of us, one that will likely visit us at least once or twice throughout our lifetimes. Depression affects each of us in different ways, and the effects depend on a variety of factors. Genetics, specific personality traits, biochemistry and certain environment factors such as socioeconomic status, cementation in the poverty cycle, and environments where neglect and abuse are prevalent can all contribute to the development of depression symptoms.

As a first responder, you should be aware that depression is something you will encounter regularly. It is important for you to understand that depression is treatable, so that you can reassure the person suffering with the mental health emergency that things will be alright—there *is* hope and there *is* help.

WHAT DOES DEPRESSION LOOK LIKE IN A MENTAL HEALTH EMERGENCY?

- Hollowness; feeling empty inside

- Feeling sad and showing sorrow

- Fatigue and extreme tiredness, often a residual from physical exertion and overall mental health

- Loss of energy or lower sustained physical and mental activities

- Loss of interest in activities that were once fun

- Withdrawing from hobbies and friendships

- Disruption of sleep (either getting no sleep at all or sleeping too much)

- Trouble with concentration and thinking; trouble with basic recall.

- Feelings of guilt

- Feelings of inadequacy: "I'm worthless" or "I hate myself!"

- Continued thoughts of suicide and dying

- Changes in one's eating habits (either eating too little or eating too much)

- Poor hygiene: not brushing one's teeth, not bathing, or not changing into clean clothes. (It is common for you run into people who look unkempt and disheveled; this could be a direct result of their depression.)

DISORDERS RELATED TO DEPRESSION

Seasonal Affective Disorder (SAD)

Seasonal Affective Disorder (SAD) is a type of depression that usually sets in during the winter months, and is common in parts of the world where there's limited sunlight. Individuals experiencing SAD have mood changes that mimic those of depression. SAD usually corrects itself, and symptoms improve during the changes that come with spring. Therapy lights for the home or office and vitamin D supplements are quick tactics to combat SAD.

TYPES OF DEPRESSIVE DISORDERS

When referring to specific depressive disorders, three main categories are used:

Disruptive Mood Dysregulation Disorders: Refers to a mental disorder characterized by a persistently irritable or angry mood and frequent temper outbursts that are disproportionate to the situation.

Major Depressive Disorder: A mental disorder characterized by two weeks or more of persistent "low mood." Criteria from five different categories are used to diagnose a person with major depressive disorder.

Persistent Depressive Disorder (Dysthymia): This disorder represents a consolidation of chronic major depressive disorder and dysthymic disorder. Criteria from eight different categories are used to diagnose a person with this disorder.

TREATING DEPRESSION

The good news is depression is treatable and people who seek professional mental help and who exercise can recover much more quickly. It is recommended that the individual suffering with depression seek help from a medical professional and mental health professional. In some cases, people may also need the assistance of medication management to help with brain chemistry, the most common being anti-depressants. Individual therapy and group therapy are methods that also work.

In addition to specific treatment, there are a number of options available for self-care, including:

- Exercise: i.e. yoga, martial arts, baseball, hiking, surfing, lifting weights, walking, and running

- Meditation and breathing exercises

- Priming in the morning and establishing a morning ritual (proper planning for the day that maximizes the use of your down time and plans your day properly)

- Hobbies and mindfulness activities: i.e. marksmanship, hunting, painting, and pottery

- Proper diet and nutrition (refer to the nutrition guide on page 130)

- Avoidance of drugs and alcohol

- Social supports: friends, family, support groups and clergy

- Complete an Advanced Directive when you are well, outlining what happens to you when you are in a mental health crisis and what steps work, to assist you in restoring wellness.

CHAPTER 8

Somatic Symptoms

SOMATIC SYMPTOMS ARE when people have a strong focus on their physical symptoms which, in some cases, may occur without a direct physical cause. This focus can manifest as anxiety or excessive thoughts, feelings, and behaviors that relate to the physical symptoms that they are experiencing. These create a great amount of distress, which in turn becomes a major disruption to their quality of life. The focus is often placed on pain in the body, shortness of breath, and perceived weakness in the body.

It is important to note that the person is not faking their illness or exaggerating their experience. They *are* indeed experiencing some symptoms of physical ailment, though the symptoms may or may not be associated with a diagnosable medical condition or illness. These complaints usually need a prolonged period before a psychiatrist can weigh in and provide professional mental health support. Often, a person will be seen by a primary physician many times, with only superficial results.

TREATMENT FOR SOMATIC SYMPTOMS

It is recommended that an individual presenting with somatic symptoms be seen by a mental health professional, particularly if symptoms include obsessive ongoing thoughts about the physical symptoms and their physical causes. It is hard to get a person to recognize these concerns as being mental health issues and often they only want to be seen by their primary medical doctor or medical facilities, even going so far as to make multiple visits to the emergency room of a hospital or emergency outpatient facility.

It is also recommended that the person receive psychotherapy to disrupt and change their thinking patterns, to better target the behaviors that consume their psychical thoughts and symptoms. Activities like mindfulness, meditation, breathing and yoga are a great complement to talk therapy, and can help address the body's stress and its ability to properly deal with the pain. If the person is experiencing anxiety and depression because of the obsessive and excessive thoughts, appropriate medication may be recommended by a professional.

CHAPTER 9

Personality Disorders

THE DSM-5 DESCRIBES a personality disorder as "a way of thinking, feeling and behaving that deviates from the expectations of culture, causes distress or problems functioning, and lasts over time" (American Psychiatric Association, 2013). Personality disorders can be difficult to manage at times, and can easily complicate matters when you are tending to a mental health emergency.

TYPES OF PERSONALITY DISORDERS

The American Psychiatric Association groups personality disorders into categories called "clusters":

CLUSTER A: ODD OR ECCENTRIC BEHAVIOR
Paranoid Personality Disorder
Persons suffering from paranoid personality disorder will demonstrate a pronounced distrust of others. They will be suspicious of people and will not confide in or develop relation-

ships with others. When dealing with someone you believe is suffering from this disorder, be sure to give the person space and time to process what is going on. Use silence to your advantage when communicating, and build trust by using empathy.

Schizoid Personality Disorder

Persons with schizoid personality disorder show a pattern of detachment from social relationships and have a limited range of emotional expression. They are indifferent to praise or criticism from others, and will invariably choose solitary activities over working with a group. Avoid using praise and platitudes when speaking with these individuals. Instead, exercise empathy, active listening and silence.

Schizotypal Personality Disorder

Persons with schizotypal personality disorder exhibit a pattern of acute discomfort in close relationships, distortions in thinking and perception, and eccentric behavior. A person with schizotypal personality disorder may have odd beliefs or "magical thinking," odd or peculiar behavior or speech, or may incorrectly attribute meanings to events.

Avoid using praise and platitudes when speaking with these individuals. Exercise empathy, active listening and silence.

CLUSTER B: DRAMATIC, EMOTIONAL OR ERRATIC BEHAVIOR

Antisocial Personality Disorder

While the labels "psychopath," "sociopath," and "antisocial personality disorder" have been used interchangeably, the core of the complaint is when a person demonstrates a pattern of disregarding or violating the rights of others. A person with antisocial personality disorder may not conform to social norms, may repeatedly lie or deceive others, lack remorse or may act impulsively. They have a propensity to break all the rules. A poor marriage or work record and criminal history are common with these individuals.

People with antisocial personality disorders are difficult to deal with and they usually have a hard time coming to grips with their illness. When they get referred to appropriate professional mental health help, they are known to "go through the motions," without taking their treatment seriously, and often they find themselves in an endless cycle. When helping these people through a crisis, understand that they may not acknowledge any wrongdoing on their part. Continue using your empathy and active listening skills until the situation resolves itself.

Borderline Personality Disorder

An individual with borderline personality disorder displays a pattern of instability in personal relationships, emotional response, self-image and impulsivity. A person with borderline personality disorder may go to great lengths to avoid abandonment (real or perceived), have recurrent suicidal behavior, and display inappropriate or intense anger. Without a core identity, impulsivity grabs a hold of these individuals, making them prone to excess in areas like hyper-sexual activity, shopping, drinking, drugs and extreme activities like racing cars and sky-diving. Their crises may include gambling addictions, sexually transmitted diseases from unprotected sex, marital problems, divorce, and battles with drugs and alcohol.

Remember that borderline personality disorder individuals

are quick to anger, which can show itself with self-deprecation, cynicism, or sardonic behavior that can escalate to an aggressive state. Please refer to Chapter 20 on de-escalation for special tactics.

Histrionic Personality Disorder

Once known as "dramatic and erratic," histrionic personality disorder describes individuals with a pattern of excessive emotions and attention seeking behaviors. A person with histrionic personality disorder may be uncomfortable when he/she is not the center of attention, and may consistently use their physical appearance to draw attention or show rapidly shifting or exaggerated emotions. These individuals may vacillate from day to day, or even from moment to moment. They are also known to use seductive behaviors to grab attention and they are quick to throw a temper tantrum when they feel it is necessary.

Persons with histrionic personality disorder can also exhibit some very positive qualities and traits; they can be very extroverted, outgoing and assertive. Per Oldham and Morris (Oldham, Morris, 1995) histrionics are "idea people;" they are often creative, artsy people. Be careful to recognize their inherent fear of abandonment and rejection by those around them. They may even have an underlying fear that you will abandon them in your pursuit to assist in their crisis. Use your empathy and active listening skills to show you are concerned, listening and that you are there to help assist them through their crisis.

Narcissistic Personality Disorder

The word "narcissist," derived from the handsome and gregarious Narcissus of Greek legend who was in love with his own reflection, describes a pattern of need for admiration and a lack of empathy for others. Narcissists usually have a grandiose sense of self-importance, a sense of entitlement; they take advantage of others and/or lack empathy. Do not expect the narcissist to behave in a rational or cooperative way.

Don't get stuck in their charm. Stick to *your* agenda and protocol(s) and not theirs. Solicit their assistance in the crisis and make them understand that there are personal rewards attached to helping the crisis or emergency. Keep them engaged, the center of attention, and express that you value their skills. This will enable you to better gain their trust. When you are establishing rapport with the individual, remember to find areas of common ground.

CLUSTER C: ANXIOUS OR FEARFUL BEHAVIOR

Avoidant Personality Disorder

The person exhibits a pattern of social inhibition, feelings of inadequacy and extreme sensitivity to criticism. A person with avoidant personality disorder may be unwilling to get involved with people unless they are certain they will be liked. They view themselves as being inferior or socially inept. Preoccupation with oneself becomes a barrier to communicating.

Dependent Personality Disorder

Person with dependent personality disorder exhibit a pattern of needing to be taken care of. Known for submissive and clingy behavior, the person usually has difficulty making decisions about their personal daily activities.

Obsessive Compulsive Personality Disorder

A pervasive pattern of preoccupation with orderliness, perfectiveness, and mental and interpersonal control, at the expensive of flexibility, openness, and efficiency. Obsessive compulsive personality disorder tends to manifest in early adulthood.

TREATMENT FOR PERSONALITY DISORDERS

What are the treatments for personality disorders? In truth, there *are* no specific treatments recommended for emergency situations dealing with personality disorders, as they are very difficult to discern. If some of these types of behavior start to surface, be cognizant of your own actions and rely on trained medical professionals.

People who are diagnosed with these types of personality disorders should try to avoid substances such as drugs and alcohol, as these can worsen their symptoms. Self-management and good self-care, archiving behaviors in a journal for heightened self-awareness, and the help of socialization, group therapy and support activities are all beneficial for managing symptoms and increasing one's quality of life.

Dialectical behavioral therapy, which was first designed to treat suicidal borderline personality disorders, is currently considered the gold standard of care for this population.

CHAPTER 10

Obsessive-Compulsive Behaviors

OBSESSIVE-COMPULSIVE DISORDER (OCD) describes a condition where a person becomes trapped in a cycle of obsessions and compulsions. Obsessions are intrusive thoughts, images or urges that are unwanted and which trigger intense feelings of distress. Compulsions are the resulting behavior the person engages in to get rid of their obsessions, and to decrease their feelings of distress.

Examples of OCD include mental compulsions, consuming thoughts and ideas, excessive cleaning, repeating actions, checking and rechecking, and constantly ordering and arranging aspects of their life or environment.

TYPES OF OBSESSIVE-COMPULSIVE DISORDERS

Body Dysmorphic Disorder

The individual is preoccupied with one or more perceived defects or flaws in their physical appearance, which they believe make them look ugly, unattractive, abnormal, or deformed. These preoccupations are intrusive, unwanted, time-consuming (on average 3–8 hours a day) and usually difficult to resist or control.

Hoarding Disorder

Hoarding disorder is when a person has an extreme difficulty discarding possessions (usually those with no extrinsic value), and as a result begins to "hoard" the items in their home or dwelling. This repeated, obsessive focus on collection often affects individuals emotionally, physically, socially, financially and legally. The person's distress comes from the thought of parting with the items, so these things start to consume their space.

First responders entering a hoarding environment should exercise extreme safety precautions. It may be unsafe to breathe, hard to walk freely, or be difficult to navigate. You also have the threat of rodents running about. Having some pioneer gear (gloves, breathing masks, axes, shovels, rakes) on your person or vehicle could be a big help, as there may be a time where you have to shovel your way to the victim in the mental health crisis.

After the crisis resolves, the only quick solution would be to recommend a "muck out," where the person's dwelling is purged of all unnecessary items to address public health concerns. For this procedure, it is recommended that you enlist the aid of the appropriate mental health professionals, who can offer an intensive and concentrated mental health treatment.

Skin Picking Disorder (Excoriation Disorder)
Excessive skin picking (excoriation) is the recurrent skin picking in skin lesions and acne regions, and is classified under OCD. You may notice lesions on some people who suffer from this disorder; they may also have scabs and active acne regions on their body.

This behavior can cause distress and impairment in daily living, social and occupational settings. You can recommend good local medical and mental health resources in your community, along with support groups and treatment literature.

Hair Pulling Disorder (Trichotillomania)
Hair pulling disorder describes the impulsive desire to pick, pull, and pluck hair follicles excessively from the body. You may notice missing patches in the person's hair, beard, eyebrows, eyelashes, and underarms.

TREATMENT FOR OBSESSIVE-COMPULSIVE DISORDER

Cognitive Behavioral Therapy (CBT)
Cognitive Behavioral Therapy (CBT) is considered the most efficient therapy in terms of results obtained. It is based upon the premise that our thoughts cause our feelings and behaviors, not external things like people, situations or events. The benefit to this model is that we can change the way we think to feel or act better, even if the situation does not change.

Dialectical Behavior Therapy

Dialectical Behavior Therapy is effective at helping people manage overwhelming emotions. Research shows that DBT strengthens a person's ability to handle distress without losing control or acting destructively.

Psychotherapy

Psychotherapy is designed to disrupt or change thinking patterns to better target the behaviors that consume psychical thoughts and symptoms. Activities like mindfulness, meditation, breathing and yoga are a great complement to talk therapy, and can help address the body's stress and its ability to properly deal with OCD.

CHAPTER 11

Substance Use Disorders

HE TERM "SUBSTANCE abuse" refers to the taking of large, unnecessary amounts of a substance to achieve heightened levels of the substance's effects. The most common substance use disorders first responders will see, both on the streets and in the homes of the public, are alcohol and opioid abuse. Many people with substance use disorders want to cut down and quit, yet they struggle. Often, many areas of their personal life begin to suffer because of their use. Their relationships begin to suffer at home, school and work. They may isolate or lose key relationships.

As a first responder, it will be very common to find co-morbidity when dealing with individuals struggling with substance abuse. Co-morbidity means that the individual will have a substance use disorder coupled with a mental health illness, which they may be trying to self-medicate by using and abusing their substance of choice. The person may exhibit signs of personal debt, such as the selling of personal effects.

The following are risk factors that can contribute to the development of a substance use disorder:

- Availability and tolerance of the substance in society; i.e., cocktails being offered at social gatherings, bars, restaurants, and liquor stores; marijuana becoming recreationally legal in some states

- Genetic predisposition

- Sensitivity to the substance

- Learned behaviors, including behaviors learned while growing and the messages received from the immediate environment

- Other mental health problems

Let us state for the record that just because someone uses alcohol or drugs it does not mean that person has a substance use *disorder*. Substance use disorders (or SUDs) include the abuse and/or dependence on alcohol or drugs and their effects to "balance" or impede on school, work, home life, relationships, and legal problems. The dependence on and abuse of these substances leads to problems at home or work, with personal and professional relationships, and may also cause severe damage to one's health. Substance use disorders can co-occur with almost any mental illness, and people with anxiety or mood disorders are two to three times more likely to have a substance use disorder.

Common substances involved in substance use disorders include:

- Marijuana (and synthetic marijuana), including edibles

- Heroin (and other opioids/pain killers/prescription medications)

- Sedatives and tranquilizers (reduces irritability)

- Cocaine

- Amphetamines (stimulant)

- Methamphetamines (stimulant, sometimes used to treat ADHD and weight loss)

- Ecstasy and other hallucinogens

- "Bath salts," a synthetic drug in crystal form

- Inhalants (aerosols, gases, and paint)

- Tobacco

- Alcohol

SYMPTOMS OF SUBSTANCE USE DEPENDENCE

Over time, an individual will feel the need for increased amounts of a substance, as they build up a tolerance. Since withdrawal symptoms are difficult to deal with, the temptation to increase one's usage is strong. Even if a person should try to quit using a substance, the withdrawal symptoms alone could be enough to rope them back into using.

Another symptom is the large amount of time and energy a person will spend trying to obtain their substance of choice, not to mention the time lost while using it and recovering from its effects. The substance starts to take priority over one's other responsibilities, forcing the person to prioritize their using around personal and important life events.

Perhaps worst of all, the person will be aware of the consequences of substance abuse, but will keep on with the behaviors and continue using, knowing full well the risks they run. This in turn contributes to a growing sense of shame, guilt or low emotional value of one's self, which may cause them to use the substance anyway, just to escape from those feelings feel comfortable in their own skin, which may cause them to use the substance anyway, just to escape from those emotions (take out feelings) and feel comfortable in their own skin.

So, as a first responder, what signs should you look for? Some common signs with active users include:

- Pupils that are constricted, usually a sign that the person is intoxicated

- Opioid users may exhibit signs of dry "cotton" mouth, and will voice problems about constipation and bowel movements

- Women will share that they are having disruptions or irregular menstrual cycles (periods)

- Visible rawness in the person's nasal cavity

TYPES OF SUBSTANCE USE DISORDERS

Alcohol

In the United States, moderate drinking is categorized as consuming up to two drinks per day for men and one drink per day for women. Any consumption of five drinks or more on the same occasion constitutes the definition of binge drinking as put forward by the Substance Abuse and Mental Health Administration (SAMSA). SAMSA also categorizes the drinking behavior of five drinks per day for a period of five days or more in the past thirty days as "heavy drinking." The unrestrained and excessive consumption of alcohol over time places someone's physical and mental health at risk and puts an individual at risk for greater safety concern.

Marijuana

Marijuana is a mind-altering drug that is a mixture of dried leaves, seeds, stems and flowers of the hemp plant. The main active chemical ingredient of marijuana is delta-9-tetrahydro-cannabinol (THC), the effect of which varies by individual and depends on the level of THC contained. The level of THC in marijuana continues to increase as more and more potent varieties are bred. Marijuana use can interfere with school and work performance.

Marijuana is the most commonly used substance (after alcohol and tobacco) in the United States. As more and more states make marijuana use legal for recreational use, more and more people are beginning to use it in many forms and the prevalence of marijuana use amongst younger people is beginning to grow.

Some of the concerns in regards to the effects of marijuana use include impaired thinking and motor function, which involves the fine use of muscles in the body (include the tongue, lips, fingers, toes, wrists, legs, arms, and the ability to crawl, walk and jump). Long term use of marijuana can create respiratory issues, and even increases the likelihood of developing certain cancers. Younger people are more susceptible to developing mental illness with heavy use and in some cases they will experience irritability, restlessness, paranoia, anxiousness, nervousness, anger, depression and even psychosis.

Amphetamines/Methamphetamines

Amphetamines belong to the stimulant category of drugs and have the effect of temporarily increasing energy and producing the appearance of a heightened mental awareness. The formal use of the drug is for attention deficit hyperactivity disorder (known as ADHD), but amphetamines are also used to treat other medical conditions such as obesity and narcolepsy. Recreationally, it is used for euphoria and libido.

High doses of these drugs can lead to anxiety, paranoia, aggression and psychotic symptoms. As the effects wear off, a person may experience concerning issues with irritability, agitation, substance and food cravings, with increased appetite and/or sleeplessness. Amphetamines come in many forms such as powder, tablets, capsules, crystals or liquid.

Methamphetamines are like amphetamines in their chemical structure, but have a stronger effect on the brain, with symptoms lasting up to eight hours. After the substance takes hold, a state of agitation results that can lead to violent behaviors. Some prescription drugs are comprised of the amphetamine structure and are intended to address attention-deficit/hyperactivity disorder and other medical conditions.

Cocaine

Cocaine is a powerful stimulant drug derived from the leaves of a coca plant that is native to South America. Cocaine is snorted through the nose, rubbed on gums, injected and smoked. Cocaine is the most commonly abused illicit drug in North America, followed by marijuana and heroin. The substance increases the natural levels of dopamine and its short-term effects create extreme happiness, mental alertness, paranoia (extreme distrust for others), irritability and hypersensitivity to sights, sounds and touch with an increased energy.

Cocaine is the most common illegal drug you will see as a first responder. Cocaine's physical symptoms may include enlarged pupils, profuse sweating, and an accelerated heartbeat, as well as raised blood pressure and body temperature. Mentally, the individual will sometimes lose contact with reality when they are "high" and may appear to be agitated. Their mood may also be elevated with intense happiness. The effects can come on very quickly after use and range anywhere from minutes to up to an hour and half. Cocaine is an addictive substance with a propensity for drug dependence because its reward activity is closely linked to the brain's natural function. Cocaine plays on the brain's dopamine, serotonin, and norepinephrine by inhibiting their reuptake.

Heroin

Heroin is an opioid drug. Heroin is synthesized from morphine, a substance extracted from an opium poppy plant. Heroin appears in several forms and different colors, such as white, brown and black tar. A large percentage of individuals who use heroin become dependent on it. These substances cause drug seeking behavior and habitual relapse(s). The substance can be made to be injected with a needle, smoked or inhaled by sniffing/snorting through the nose. Heroin overdoses usually involve hypoxia (suppression of oxygen making its way to the brain).

Inhalants

Known by their nicknames of "poppers," "sniffles," and "whippets," inhalants are breathable vapors from toxic chemical substances that are found in a multitude of household products, such as glues, gasoline, paint thinners, paints, and nitrous oxide. Young people are more inclined to abuse these substances because of their inexpensive nature and their availability. Often, people become dependent on inhalants if they start using them at an early age. Inhalants destroy cells in the brain, kidney, and liver.

TREATMENT FOR SUBSTANCE USE DISORDERS

When treating substance use disorders, it must be understood that shame is the biggest barrier to seeking treatment. The person must *want* to change to successfully begin the road to recovery. No amount of external persuasion will help a person overcome addiction. Understand that addiction is not the only problem; the collateral personal problems of the individual can cause damage to family, friends and colleagues. Addiction spares no group, race, religion, economic class, gender, sexual orientation, level of success, or family structure. Before deciding on a treatment, understanding the age and extent of the addiction is imperative, along with co-occurring mental health disorders. (After all, over one-third of alcohol abusers and half of drug abusers have a diagnosable mental health disorder.)

A few factors in considering treatment options are the setting, modality, available providers and duration. Settings are where the service is provided and include outpatient (ambulatory), residential (inpatient), or community facilities (churches or community centers). Modality is how the service will be managed, such as a treatment team approach, which would include counselors, nurses, social workers, psychologists, psychiatrists; self-help treatment approaches, utilizing individual counseling with treatment models such as Cognitive Behavioral Therapy, Dialectal Behavioral Therapy, Trauma Related Therapy, and group therapy; and pharmacology.

Properly investigating providers who provide addiction treatment is essential to the individual success of each person. There are different categories of clinicians and non-clinicians who provide addiction treatment. There are also 12-step programs, which help the individual every step of the way, and addiction counselors, who assist the individual in managing their addiction (along with related mental health issues). Duration of the treatment is the most controversial section, due to the recurrent nature of addiction and the variables of each individual.

Regardless of which treatment a person chooses, one must understand that it affects each individual differently, both physically and mentally. Getting help with other primary areas of life, such as employment, family and psychological concerns, is also important to overcoming addiction. When deciding to begin substance use disorder treatment, always seek a full medical evaluation by a licensed physician.

CHAPTER 12

Psychosis

I N YOUR DAY-TO-DAY duty, you will likely hear the term "psychosis" being thrown around a lot on emergency calls. It is common to see psychosis occur in people ages 15–30, and symptoms can be triggered by a myriad of factors, such as sleep deprivation, drug use, early and advanced stages of certain physical illnesses, head injuries, and residuals from certain mental health illnesses, such as severe clinical depression, bipolar disorder and schizophrenia.

DEFINING PSYCHOSIS

It is generally understood that many factors contribute to the development of psychosis, including biochemistry, genetics, and levels of stress. The level of stress and the level of drug use in the individual may provoke psychotic symptoms in people who are susceptible. Any changes to the brain or dysfunction in the neurotransmitters may be a direct result of biological and genetic predisposition.

The common telltale signs you may come across are speech

disorders, scattered thoughts, and auditory and visual hallucinations (talking to one's self or to others that are not there, or seeing things that are not present). The Early Assessment and Support Alliance (EASA) does an excellent job of outlining the emergence of symptoms of psychosis, as the admittedly broad term applies to mental health:

"Psychotic disorders rarely emerge suddenly. Most often, the symptoms evolve and become gradually worse over a period of months or even years. Early symptoms often include cognitive and sensory changes which can cause significant disability before the illness becomes acute and is finally diagnosed. Identifying and responding appropriately to the condition early can help to get the person and their family support."

Some common symptoms of psychosis include:

- **Symptoms of reduced performance, such as:**

    + Trouble reading or understanding complex sentences

    + Trouble speaking or understanding what others are saying

    + Becoming easily confused or lost

    + Trouble in sports or other activities that used to be easy (Example: can't dribble basketball or pass to team members)

    + Attendance problems related to sleep or fearfulness

- **Changes in behavior, such as:**

    + Extreme fear for no apparent reason

    + Uncharacteristic and bizarre actions or statements

+ New, bizarre beliefs

+ Incoherent or bizarre writing

+ Extreme social withdrawal

+ Decline in appearance and hygiene

+ Dramatic changes in sleeping or eating

- **Changes in perception, including:**

    + Fear that others are trying to hurt them

    + Heightened sensitivity to sights, sounds, smells or touch

    + Making statements like, "My brain is playing tricks on me"

    + Hearing voices or sounds that others don't

    + Reporting visual changes (colors more intense, faces distorted, lines turned wavy)

    + Feeling like someone else is putting thoughts into their brain or that others are reading their thoughts

Early on, symptoms may be intermittent and the person often recognizes that something is wrong. As psychosis progresses, people lose their ability to distinguish symptoms from reality, and it becomes more difficult to have a conversation. For example, a person who has auditory hallucinations will hear voices which sound to them as loud and as real as though a person were standing right next to them, even though others don't hear it.

Complicating matters, a person whose psychosis has

progressed may not believe that other people don't hear the same voices and may not be able to integrate new information from others into their thinking.

Psychosis often comes in episodes and may involve the following phases, which may vary in duration:

- **Pre-morbid** (at-risk phase): the person does not experience symptoms, but has risk factors for developing psychosis

- **Prodromal** (becoming unwell phase): the person has some changes in emotions, motivations, thinking, perception, or behavior

- **Acute** (psychotic phase): the person is unwell, with psychotic symptoms such as delusions, hallucinations, disorganized thinking, and a reduction in ability to maintain social relationships, and/or work or study

People struggling with episodic conditions like psychosis are said to be in stages of recovery and/or relapse. Recovery is the "get well" phase, as the individual journeys to attain a level of good health and well-being. Relapse is the "back again" phase, where the person may have only one new episode, or may have additional episodes.

SYMPTOMS OF PSYCHOSIS

Changes in Thinking

During psychosis, the following changes in emotion and motivation begin to happen, which may include the following:

- Anxiety

- Irritability

- Depression

- Suspiciousness and being suspicious of people and close loved ones

- Flat, blunted, or inappropriate emotion, i.e. bursts of laughter during serious moments

- Changes in appetite and diet

- Reduced energy and motivation

The following are changes to one's thinking and perception common to psychotic episodes:

- Difficulties with attention, focus and concentration

- A sense of alteration, feeling that others are acting differently

- Odd ideas

- Unusual perception experiences, such as reduction or greater intensity of smell, sound, or color

Changes in Behavior

A person with psychosis may start to withdraw and isolate, which in turn limits their ability to maintain relationships in social settings, such as school or work. When this sort of withdrawal presents itself along with other potential symptoms it is a good indication that things may not being going well. As a first responder, it's important not to ignore or dismiss these warning signs. Do not assume that this is just a quirk of the person's character, or that it's simply the result of the person misusing drugs or alcohol, or that the symptoms will go away on their own.

The signs and symptoms of psychosis vary from person to person and can change over time, and require consideration of the individual's cultural and spiritual context. Individuals experiencing the early stages of psychosis often go undiagnosed for a year or more before receiving professional treatment. They account for a substantial portion of symptoms associated with schizophrenia, but are less prominent in other psychotic disorders.

One reason is that psychosis often develops in late childhood or adolescence and can be masked with the behaviors and emotions common to that age or younger age groups. Many young people will experience symptoms without developing psychosis, while others will eventually be diagnosed with a psychotic disorder.

SCHIZOPHRENIA SPECTRUM AND OTHER PSYCHOTIC DISORDERS

The five key factors that define psychotic disorders are Delusions, Hallucinations, Disorganized Thinking (Speech), Grossly Disorganized or Abnormal Motor Behavior (Including Catatonia) and Negative Symptoms. The following disorders present with some or all of these symptoms in some shape or form:

Schizophrenia

Contrary to popular opinion, schizophrenia does not mean split personality; rather, it is a change in mental function(s) where thoughts and perceptions become fractured and disordered, with psychosis being the main feature. The major symptoms include delusions, hallucinations, a difficulty in thinking, loss of drive, social withdrawal and blunted emotions. The presence of these negative symptoms is one of the five criteria used for diagnosis.

Schizophrenia affects 2.4 million Americans each year (roughly 1.1 percent of the U.S. population) with most people experiencing their first episode between 15–30 years of age. It affects males more often than females, and usually develops a lot earlier in men than in women. The onset of illness is usually rapid, with the symptoms developing over several weeks, though it could take a slower route and develop over several months (or even years). Most research suggests that approximately one-third of people who develop schizophrenia have only one episode and then fully recover; another third have multiple episodes but feel well in between episodes; and the final third have the illness for life.

Having a parent or sibling with schizophrenia puts one at a slightly higher risk (a 10–15 percent chance) of developing the illness themselves, but one must realize that the odds are in the favor of *not* developing it.

Other risk factors include:

- Urban living
- Moving about and migration
- Social stresses
- Marijuana use (particularly in adolescence)
- Older age of father (evidence is insubstantial, but may be due to genetic mutation and impaired sperm)
- Birth in winter or spring, as well as birth complications

Bipolar Disorder and Related Disorders

Bipolar disorder describes a condition where people have extreme mood swings, experiencing bouts of depression and bouts of mania. When an individual is on an upswing of mania they experience great excitement, over activity, euphoria and delusions.

Bipolar I and Bipolar II are classified differently, as follows:

- **Bipolar I**: This diagnosis fits the classic manic-depression state of an individual, in that neither psychosis nor a lifetime experience of major depressive disorder needs to be present for this diagnosis.

- **Bipolar II**: Requires the lifetime experience of at least one episode of major depression and one hypomanic episode classified as more than mild.

- **Cyclothymic Disorder**: This diagnosis is given to individuals who experience both hypomanic and depressive periods and have never met criteria for an episode of mania, hypomania, or major depression.

While in a manic state, a person may experience the following symptoms:

- Increased energy and over activity

- Elevated mood

- Needing less sleep than usual

- Irritability

- Rapid thinking and speech

- Lack of inhibitions

- Grandiose delusions

- Lack of insight

The person will appear to be easily excitable, overly happy and project the feeling that they are unbeatable. Often, they will stay awake for several days with little or no sleep. The person will show irritability when others don't buy into their unrealistic concepts or are unwilling to go along with their plans. A key feature of mania is talking very rapidly and changing quickly from one subject to the next. The person may also become a high risk-taker, engaging in unprotected sex, sexual jaunts, gambling, extreme sports like sky diving, racing cars and other risky situations, as well as spending of their money very liberally.

It is still not understood what the root causes of bipolar disorder are, but many have offered that having a close relative with bipolar disorder puts you at a greater risk of developing the disorder. The following are being researched as possible risk factors:

- Pregnancy and obstetric complications

- Being born in the winter or spring

- Exposure to certain social situations

- Recent stressful life events

- Recent childbirth

- Multiple sclerosis

- Traumatic brain injuries

- Gifted young children and the progression of low scores in standardized testing

Just like in schizophrenia, biochemical changes in the brain may lead to depression and mania. The time between episodes may vary greatly depending on the person. It is not unusual for people with this disorder to become psychotic during depressive or manic episodes. People with bipolar will also often abuse drugs and alcohol.

Psychotic Depression
When depression becomes too intense, it often causes psychotic symptoms where one may feel delusions of hopelessness, severe physical illness and guilt.

Schizoaffective Disorder
A condition where symptoms of a mood disorder and symptoms of schizophrenia are both present. It is often difficult for even a mental health professional to distinguish between bipolar disorder and schizophrenia/schizoaffective disorder, as the individual has symptoms of both illnesses.

Drug-Induced Psychosis
Withdrawal from and intoxication by drugs and/or alcohol can both bring on psychosis, which can appear vigorously and last for a short period, anywhere from a few hours to a few days, until the drug(s) wear off. Symptoms often include disorientation, visual hallucinations and memory problems. Please note that both legal and illegal prescriptions/medication drugs can contribute to a psychotic episode. The usual subjects include marijuana (cannabis), alcohol, cocaine, hallucinogens, amphetamine (speed), inhalants, opioids (pain relievers), sedatives, hypnotics, and anxiolytics (drugs that inhibit anxiety.)

Delusional Disorder

The key factor in a delusional disorder is the presence of one or more delusions that persist for at least one month.

The subtypes of delusions include:

Erotomanic type: The delusion that another person is in love with the individual. This person will usually hold a higher status than the individual, such as someone famous or a superior at work.

Grandiose type: The delusion of having some great talent or insight, or of having made some important discovery. This may include religious content.

Jealous type: The delusion of a partner being unfaithful. There is no cause to this delusion and is based upon incorrect inferences.

Persecutory type: The delusion of being spied on or conspired against, or fears of being poisoned, maliciously maligned or harassed, or obstructed in the pursuit of a long term goal. Small things are exaggerated. Individuals with this delusion show repeated attempts to gain satisfaction by legal or legislative action. They may resort to violence against those whom they believe are hurting them.

Somatic type: A delusion with a sensory component, the most common being a belief that an individual emits a foul odor, or that there is an infestation of insects in or on the skin, or that there is an internal parasite.

Brief Psychotic Disorder

The essential feature of this disorder is the sudden onset of at least one of the following positive symptoms: delusions, hallucinations, disorganized speech, or grossly abnormal psycho-motor behavior. The sudden onset must be within a two week timeframe between non-psychotic and psychotic behavior.

Schizophreniform Disorder

This disorder is distinguished by its difference in duration: including prodromal, active, and residual phases, schizophreniform disorder lasts at least1 month but less than 6 months.

Catatonia

There are 12 criteria for diagnosing catatonia, and for this reason it is usually diagnosed in an inpatient setting and can be present within most mental health diagnosis.

As with any diagnosis, these symptoms may be present as a side effect of a medical condition, medication, or substance use. This must be ruled out before any diagnosis is given. Do not assume a person is psychotic unless a medical evaluation has been completed and other factors are ruled out.

TREATMENT FOR PSYCHOSIS

Psychosis is a real emergency and it can take quite some time for the person to recover from their symptoms. In the case of drug-induced psychosis as result of methamphetamines, it can take up to 72 hours or more for the hallucinations and delusions to go away. Your job as a first responder is to get the person who is suffering to the appropriate professional medical help.

In a crisis or mental health emergency involving psychosis, it is possible that the individual may try to act upon a delusion or hallucination. In these cases, safely try to de-escalate the situation (please refer to Chapter xx on de-escalation tactics) and avoid anything that may further agitate or escalate the situation. Be mindful of your body language, economy and positioning—give the person enough comfortable space. If you're not able to safely de-escalate the situation, be prepared to call for assistance.

Once the mental health crisis or emergency staff arrives, make sure to relay any observations on the specifics of the person's behavior and symptoms. Explain whether there are additional people present to help. If you find the staff is dismissive of your observations, continue to advocate and seek additional professional assistance until the person receives the appropriate support.

The longer the delay between onset of psychosis and the start of treatment, the less likely it is that the person will recover. Research has shown that delay of treatment increases the individual's risk of depression and suicide, slows and delays the maturation process into adulthood, impacts relationships, and leads to poorer long-term functioning, increased use of drugs and alcohol, and undue disruptions in school or work.

As a first responder, be on the ready for extreme levels of anxiety and bouts of mania (highly elevated mood), which are common with psychosis. It is important not to trivialize what the person is seeing or hearing—what they happen to be experiencing is very real to them. If they ask you if you hear or see the unusual thoughts and experiences, it is okay to say that you aren't hearing or seeing what they are seeing, but that you understand that what they are experiencing is very real.

When communicating with an individual in the midst of a psychotic episode, use reflections and repeat back what they are telling you. You may find that they don't want to speak with you because it is too overwhelming, so make sure to find a safe place to sit down devoid of any other stimuli. This includes people, music, loud traffic and sirens. If you are tending to someone who has just been involved in a tragic event like a natural disaster, make sure they are free and clear of unsafe environments, whether it's a vehicle involved in a wreck, storm effects, groups of people, or the media trying to claw their way to the survivors for interviews. Use your common sense and find a safe, quiet place and a space free of debris. Politely remove any media from the scene or remove the person(s). Exercise patience and empathy, and use silence to your advantage.

CHAPTER 13

Suicidal Behaviors

DEFINING SUICIDE

Per the American Psychiatric Association, the second leading cause of death among people aged 15–34 is suicide, and a large percentage of suicides are a direct result of mental illness and substance use. As such, suicide constitutes a serious public health concern that you as a professional will be confronted with at one time or another during the course of your duty.

Suicidal behaviors are frequently (though not always) prefaced with subtle comments by the individual on the topic of suicide, or even outright threats about killing themselves. Often, there's a high level of consumption of alcohol or drug use present. The person may exhibit aggression and fits of rage or they may display impulsive or thrill seeking behavior. The withdrawal of others may have brought them to this point. A drastic change in mood from anger to immediate calm may also indicate a resolute decision to commit suicide. Watch for possessions that are of value to the individual being gifted to others.

TREATMENT OF SUICIDE

Your encounters with suicidal behaviors will be among the toughest parts of your job and it will require the culmination of the knowledge, training, and life experiences you've acquired, all to help save a life. The risk of suicide can turn a little emergency call into a big psychiatric crisis. Your immediate responsibility is to keep yourself, your team and the person in the mental health emergency safe. The next step is to immediately place the individual in the care of a medical or mental health professional. A quick go-to may be a crisis respite facility or the emergency room of a hospital. Note that in some crisis calls, the determination of a social worker or doctor is required to approve a release. An example would be somebody with suicidal ideation (having thoughts of suicide) but who has no formal method or plan to carry out the action. A medical professional may then find it appropriate to release that person into the care of a loved one.

These emergencies will require common-sense tactics and an emphasis on personal safety. Suicidal situations can involve many different and dangerous variables, such as large suspended bridges, tall structures, poisons, fires, natural hazards and firearms. If the person is actively suicidal, try to avoid assisting on your own. Enlist the help of your team, local authorities and emergency services by calling 911 or radioing for help. That said, never leave someone who is actively suicidal alone, or in the hands of someone who is less competent than you, or a person you feel can't handle the overwhelming stress of the situation. Acknowledge the suffering person's feelings and use your best listening skills, motivational interviewing and reflective communication techniques. Repeat their frustrations and concerns back to them. Say something to the effect of: "It sounds like you've been wronged and been given a raw deal." Note that too much talking can make them uneasy and put them on edge, leading to an elevated level of aggression. If the person attempts or completes their suicidal act, call for emergency medical services and administer medical first aid.

After the emergency is resolved, psychotherapy, professional supports, self-help and medications will be a good source of treatment to reduce the behaviors and thoughts around suicide.

> If you or anyone you know is experiencing a mental health emergency and is in need of immediate support and attention, call the National Suicide Prevention Line at **1-800-273-8255.** Trained crisis workers are available to help, 24 hours a day.

CHAPTER 14

Trauma and Stress Related Disorders

DEFINING TRAUMA AND TRAUMATIC EVENTS

A trauma is defined as any distressing or disturbing experience a person has, usually as a direct response to a traumatic event. Any incident experienced by a person that is perceived to be traumatic (i.e., emotionally disturbing or distressing) is considered a traumatic event. These events include car accidents, assaults (including verbal, physical and sexual), family violence, mugging, robberies and/or witnessing something gruesome or unsettling. Traumatic events also include experiences seen in combat, such as witnessing terrorist attacks or public mass shootings, and severe weather events, such as earthquakes, tsunamis, floods and forest fires.

The realistic benefits of using mental health emergency training directly after a major traumatic event are dubious at best. It is important to realize that traumatic events are not a singular incident involving a single individual; mental health emergency tactics should only be administered in cases of traumatic events when the first responder is made aware of a specific mental emergency.

Circumstances where this might be the case include the following:

- Recurring trauma, such as:

    + Sexual, physical or emotional abuse

    + Torture: i.e. being forced to starve, do hard labor, and being forced in uncomfortable positions

    + Bullying in the school or workplace and cyber-bullying online in social media

- Memories of a traumatic event which suddenly or unexpectedly return weeks, months, or even years afterwards, which can lead to a level of distress and discomfort

It is also important to note that people differ in how they react to traumatic events. One person may perceive an event as deeply traumatic, while another does not, and certain types of traumas affect some individuals more than others. A history of trauma may make some people more susceptible to later traumatic events, while others show more resiliency.

TYPES OF TRAUMATIC AND STRESS-RELATED DISORDERS

Post-Traumatic Stress Disorder (PTSD)

Post-traumatic stress disorder (PTSD) is commonly associated with military members and veterans who experienced traumatic events during combat. When you hear "fight or flight" responses described, these are common responses to this disorder. A person suffering with PTSD will exhibit anxiousness and fear, even though there is no visible danger present. PTSD can affect anyone, and its usual causes include combat, terrorism, natural threats, divorce, car accidents, abandonment, witnessing death, death of a loved one, domestic abuse, sexual assault and rape.

As a first responder treating someone with PTSD, understand that the person may have dissociative reactions (essentially "flashbacks") where the person relives the trauma repeatedly. Signs of this include sweating profusely and having frightening thoughts that dominate their mental state. Such reactions occur on a continuum, the most extreme of which is a complete loss of awareness of one's present surroundings.

Reactive Attachment Disorder (RAD)

Reactive attachment disorder (RAD) is a disorder found in a small percentage of children, and deals with specific attachments that happen prior to age five. These children often experience emotional, physical and sexual abuse. This in turn makes it difficult for a young person to establish "normal" and loving relationships. When treating someone you believe is suffering from RAD, remember to exercise your empathy and quick listening skills. These youths rarely seek or respond to comfort when distressed.

TREATING TRAUMA

As a first responder, what should your priority be after a traumatic event?

- Find out what additional emergency help will be on the scene to assist you and your team. Tap the talent of volunteers, groups, agencies and the assistance of state and federal aid workers.

- As with any mental health emergency encounter, make sure to respect the comfort and dignity of the person you are helping. Offer a blanket or coat to cover them, and ask bystanders or media to move out of the way. Try not to appear anxious, impatient, or rushed. Show them with your body language that you are here to help and that you will assist through this crisis.

- Give truthful information. If you don't have any answers, learn to be comfortable saying, "I don't know, but I will try and find out and get back to you with an answer." Provide information and resources as they become available. However, do not provide information that the person does not want or need to hear, as this can trigger recent memories of their experience and be very traumatic for them.

- Establish rapport with the individual or individuals. Remember, up to 75 percent of managing a trauma is the relationship you build with the individual.

Please note: When practicing mental health emergency training during or immediately after a traumatic event, you must ensure your own safety prior to offering anyone help. Check for potential dangers; canvas the area for weapons, fire, debris, or other individuals who may become aggressive or a threat, before deciding to approach and offer help to the person in a mental health crisis.

If you are meeting the person in need for the first time, introduce yourself and explain why you are approaching. Ask the person their name, and use it while you are speaking to them; this can help you quickly build rapport with that person. Make sure that you remain calm and take that person to a safe, quiet location to remove them from any immediate danger, as well as to give them some privacy. If the person is injured physically, it is important to get them the appropriate medical treatment; use medical first aid until emergency medical help arrives. Even if the person seems to be physically unhurt, watch for changes in their physical and mental state and be prepared to seek medical assistance if necessary. Be aware that the person may have internal injuries that reveal themselves slowly or which may not be evident at all when you take your first glance, so keep your eyes peeled for any subtle hints or evidence of sudden disorientation.

Determine the person's immediate needs for food, water, clothing and shelter. If there are other emergency first responders on the scene, leverage those resources to assess and assist, and allow the other professionals to support in their own capacity. Remember, as a first responder you aren't responsible to do it all.

If you are approaching a person who is a victim of an assault, keep in mind that there's a chance you will be interacting with law enforcement. Forensic evidence will need to be collected from skin and clothing, including bodily fluids, so it is best to help preserve any evidence by placing clothing into a bag. Advise the individual not to take a shower until a forensic exam is completed. That said, please realize that you can't force someone to do anything they don't want to do. In addition, do not make any promises you cannot keep (for example, promising them they will be home soon).

When speaking to a person in a mental health emergency after they have just experienced a traumatic event, it is important to be genuine. Actively listen, show empathy and ask if you may help that person. Speak clearly and use simple language; don't be afraid to repeat yourself and simplify your message when needed. Please realize that behavior such as irritability, bad temper, and withdrawal may be a response to the trauma, not to your approach.

Others may not show any emotions or signs of grief; for some, it may even be culturally inappropriate for them to do so. Some individuals may feel compelled to relay the series of events repeatedly to you, like a broken record. In these instances, you must exercise patience and your active listening skills. Avoid saying things like, "You should be glad you're alive," or, "Calm down," or, "Don't cry." Some people might feel survivor's guilt, thinking that it's unfair that another person died or was injured while they survived. Providing support in these cases can come in the form of offering that person a glass of water, having a cup of coffee with that person, or even giving them a hug (if they are comfortable with that level of contact). On that note, it is always a good idea to ask before placing a hand on someone's shoulder or providing them with a hug.

Never assume that the person will voice their concerns of their own volition. Encourage that person to speak up and tell others when they need something. Have them identify sources of support and the people in their life that can be relied on, but also understand that person's need to be alone at times.

Encourage them to get plenty of rest and engage in activities that make them feel good, like bubble baths, exercising or watching their favorite television shows or sports teams. Allow them to think of coping strategies and defense mechanisms that have helped in the past and encourage them to spend time in places that are comfortable and safe for them. It is important to discourage excessive working, use of recreational drugs, alcohol or other self-destructive activities, as these are all negative coping strategies.

The person may experience sudden and unexpected memories, recalling vivid details of the traumatic event. They may not feel comfortable sharing the details of the event with you; however, when it appears the person might be getting overwhelmed, make sure to recommend that they seek out some form of support, including professional help. Offer your support by providing local resources and contact numbers (these should be kept readily available in your work notebook or journal). Advise them that if they are not comfortable with your recommendations, they have the right to go and see other professionals. Help them understand that they must be an advocate for their own care. If the person refuses to seek care and becomes suicidal, it is permissible to seek professional help for that person on their behalf. This is important information to pass on to the friends and family members of the individual.

The person should resume normal functioning after about four weeks or so. You must encourage professional help if any of the following continue to linger:

- They are very fearful and become easily upset

- They feel unable to escape the intense, ongoing feelings of distress

- They withdraw from friends, family and very important relationships begin to suffer

- They feel cagey, cautious and suspicious

- They have trauma-related nightmares

- They are unable to stop thinking about the trauma

- They are unable to enjoy their daily life activities

- They have post-traumatic symptoms that are barriers to daily activities and reliving certain experiences and people can place them right back in the cycle

As a first responder, you may argue that this is a lot of territory to cover, and in truth, you may not even scratch the surface in your discussion with the individual in the emergency. Regardless, it's a good idea to have a grasp of these tactics in case the need arises.

CHAPTER 15

Self-Injury

SELF-INJURY AND SELF-HARM is behavior that is closely linked to mental illness. It describes a condition where someone hurts themselves on purpose, by way of a knife, burning by flame, pulling and plucking hair, picking at their skin or open wounds, or other similar behaviors. The point where self-injury becomes a diagnosable condition is when an individual has engaged in intentional self-injury for more than five days out of the last year. What distinguishes this from suicidal thoughts or tendencies is the absence of suicide attempts, and whether the act itself is likely to result in death.

Typically, these behaviors come about due to the individual having poor or ineffective coping mechanisms. When someone hurts themselves or thinks about hurting themselves, it is a sign of emotional distress. They are the result of unseen battle wounds which hinder their ability to function in their day-to-day lives as they try to keep their injurious behaviors secret. These individuals will usually hide their cuts and scrapes with bandages or clothing.

TREATING SELF-INJURY

Make sure to talk to the person and find out what is bothering them. Don't draw too much attention to the person's sores or cuts if they aren't new. If the cuts or burns or self-injuring behavior is new, make sure that they receive the appropriate medical attention and get them to appropriate professional medical help, be it a doctor's office or an emergency room, as soon as possible. Understand that you must be discreet with this person's issue, as they are likely to be feeling a lot of shame.

CHAPTER 16

Eating Disorders

DEFINING EATING DISORDERS

Eating disorders affect individuals in several ways. Common behaviors include a preoccupation with one's appearance, extreme shifts in weight and overconsumption of food. These habits will start affecting one's quality of life greatly the longer they go on.

Eating disorders are more common in women than men. The combination of conditions in one's eating disorder can cause great physical and emotional strain on the individual and, if the disorders go untreated they can lead to serious physical harm to the body, including death.

TYPES OF EATING DISORDERS

Anorexia Nervosa

This is a mental health disorder wherein the individual denies themselves food. They will refuse to eat and if they do consume food it is in very small amounts. The individual may also practice purging and extreme exercise methods.

Bulimia Nervosa

Bulimia nervosa (or bulimia) describes recurrent episodes of binge eating (consuming large amounts of food) followed by self-induced vomiting, the use of laxatives, fasting and hyper-exercising routines. Individuals may also display an obsessive focus on continued self-validation of their body composition.

Binge Eating Disorder (BED)

Binge eating disorder describes recurrent episodes of binge eating (eating more than normal), especially consuming large amounts of food when not feeling physically hungry. Individuals may display a marked preference for consuming food alone because they are embarrassed by their behavior. In contrast to bulimia, no purging takes place.

PICA

PICA describes the eating of non-food and non-nutritive substances for a period of over one month. People with this disorder ingest items that can be found lying on the ground and they may have future medical concerns related to consuming items that cannot be digested.

TREATMENT FOR EATING DISORDERS

Eating disorders are a result of combined mental health issues, and therefore most professionals refer individuals to clinics which have a focus on and specialize in this specific type of treatment. Clinics treating these disorders focus on the mental health as well as the deteriorated physical condition of the individual due to lagging nutritional deficits causing major organs of the body to not function properly. The nature of treatment depends on the level of deterioration of bodily functions. There are times when a hospital stay will be required to stabilize the patient before any mental health treatment begins. Always ensure a medical health professional oversees any treatment concerning eating disorders.

PART III

Getting Ahead of a Mental Health Crisis

CHAPTER 17

Determining a Person's Needs

FIRST RESPONDERS RELY on extensive knowledge, approved tactics and previously established protocols to be able to assist someone in a mental health emergency. They also understand that following guidelines is necessary to figure out what each person needs assistance with. As first responder, being able to quickly and accurately assess a situation, determine the necessary care and put plans into action is paramount.

The following are a few guidelines that should help you in ascertaining what aid the individual or individuals in a mental emergency require:

- Understand that you shouldn't make promises to a person in a mental health emergency that you can't keep. For example, you cannot promise to keep a matter confidential if the person is at risk of harming themselves or others.

- When a person represents a harm to themselves or others, it is time to call law enforcement and emergency services.

- When a person is actively suicidal, self-injuring or is suffering from the side effects of or withdrawal from substance use, you must take swift action and get them to the next level of care (immediate medical emergency medical treatment).

- If the person has not slept or eaten in several days because a mental health condition, you must get that person to a hospital, particularly when it has resulted in a cessation of self-care.

- If the person is experiencing severe mania, prolonged psychosis, or severe depression symptoms, you should assist in getting them to a hospital.

- Keep the person's dignity intact. Make them feel comfortable and safe while you carry out your duties. This will go a long way towards building rapport, and will be the secret to your effectiveness during emergencies.

- Find out what the person feels their strengths are and use them to support their recovery.

NEVER ASSUME

Assuming when responding to a mental health emergency will only complicate matters and make things worse. Do not assume certain mental illnesses and diagnoses will lead to certain outcomes. Do not assume that the person you are tending to in a car accident, natural disaster, or other life threatening event is traumatized. The information in this book is intended to expand your knowledge base and give you a certain level of context and comfort. You are not to play therapist or act in ways you aren't qualified to. It isn't your prerogative to *solve* the mental health problem.

Avoid pathologizing what you and your team may or may not be seeing. When reporting to other professionals, keep the information clear, concise and free of editorializing. Make sure to stick to the facts; do not hypothesize or speculate as to what will happen next. Refrain from providing any additional information about mental illness; rather, use this to your advantage

CHAPTER 18

Support

THE SAD TRUTH is that mental health concerns can show up before, during and after emergency events. They can be a direct result of the situation at hand or they can be unrelated, the result of a previously existing condition.

For that reason, the first responder's job during a mental health emergency is to reduce distress, promote adaptive functioning and avoid eliciting traumatic feelings or experiences that may exacerbate what the person is dealing with. This is what it means to provide the person in the mental health emergency with support.

Support means grabbing just enough facts and observations to aid and assist. It is not your job or your place to provide full blown mental health treatment. First responders are the front line and usually the first point of contact in an emergency, and so it is important that you address the immediate needs of the suffering individual. Making sure the person is safe, comfortable, and cared for should be your primary focus. Embracing compassion is a key ingredient. During your first contact and any further engagement, use the same tools when responding to a physical medical emergency. Think of stabilization, safety, comfort, rapid information and fact gathering and assisting with coping mechanisms in the moment (like breathing techniques and rest) as your primary function.

When providing support, be sure to communicate in the simplest of ways, remaining clear and concise. Speak slowly and keep the cadence of your sentences short. When speaking to a young person it may be a good idea to crouch down or sit where you can have mirroring body language and level eye contact. (Use your best judgment, as this may be seen as patronizing by a young person.) When working with older people, be sensitive to age impairments, but don't ever assume limitations or impairments. Avoid first responder, medical or mental health acronyms and jargon. When the individual in crisis is talking, be prepared to truly listen to that person. Validate the positives of what the individual has done up until that point and focus on their strengths. Always, always remain positive. Focus on their needs and try to anticipate next action steps to get them some help. It is important to stay in the moment, as a person suffering with mental health will be dialed into someone else's body language. Your body language also must be in step with the current moment; don't appear to be frustrated, rushed or anxious, as this will make your job more difficult.

FIRST RESPONSE AND CONTINUING CARE

In terms of continuing care for the individual, be thinking of next action steps to link the person with the appropriate services and supports. Be cognizant of the individual and sensitive to certain identifiers and cultural sensitivities (this will develop over time as you work with different groups and get exposed to more diverse populations of people). Be humble enough to tell a person you don't understand or are not familiar with their values, diversity and cultural beliefs, but that you are interested in learning and eager to assist where appropriate.

Some people *will* continue to suffer after the initial event, but what you do in the moment can make a big impact on that person and could hopefully be the driving force for that person to seek the right treatment. By treating that person with the utmost respect, you instill in them the hope that people can go on to get better and lead happy, productive lives.

If provided the opportunity, make sure to connect the person's loved ones or family to medical and mental health resources local to the community. You may want to make clear that the individual and their family can rely on you in the future, and that you can be there as a support if needed, but be sure to explain to them your availability. Always act within the scope of your profession and make sure to establish boundaries. It is not your responsibility as a first responder to take on the role of someone's caretaker.

Continued support also means maintaining confidentiality when appropriate and necessary. Your conduct should always remain respectful and professional. This may seem like a no brainer, but can become difficult for someone who has never been verbally abused or threatened. Being stoic in your approach will allow you to ignore personal insults. Remember to never take anything personally.

In conclusion, always be respectful, show courtesy, be sensitive, patient and responsive. Allow the person to be as self-sufficient as possible. Allow them to make their own decisions regarding their care. Do not debrief the event at hand and ask them for a "rundown" of what happened. Don't forget about practical assistance, be it handing someone a glass of water, cup of coffee, food and/or a blanket during an emergency. Clearly, these are not always practical, but they can make for great tactics when trying to quickly establish rapport. If the individual is impaired or elderly, offer your arm and assistance when moving from point A to point B. If you don't know the answer to a question, don't be afraid to admit that you don't know. Tell them that you will do your best to find an answer when possible. Research local resources and have them readily available in a notebook that you carry with you. If provided the opportunity, connect them to the right social supports like family, friends, support networks and clergy if they desire.

CHAPTER 19

How to Handle Vulnerability and Build Mental Health Resiliency

MINIMIZING VULNERABILITY

Putting People at Ease

Use the following script when meeting someone for the first time:

> "Hello, my name is <u>Benjamin Franklin</u>. I am a <u>firefighter</u> with <u>the town of Philadelphia</u>. I want to check in with you and see if you are okay. Is it okay if I speak with you for a moment? What name do you prefer to go by? Please tell me what's going on."

Securing the Scene

When arriving on scene, first ensure the physical and emotional safety of all involved. For any immediate threats, make sure to engage the services of law enforcement and security services. If you are not equipped to handle safety concerns such as weapons and safety hazards, engage the service of professionals who can address this right away. Remove the individual in the mental health emergency from any unsafe spots when necessary and use your good judgement when removing liquids, sharp objects and debris from the scene. Find adequate and proper lighting in dark areas. Make sure you are visible to your other team members and ensure that your team members have good vantage points at all times.

Building Resiliency

To help build resiliency in victims, offer information on what you're about to do next and involve them in the decision-making process. Explain to them in good detail what is being done to aid and assist, and the facts that you have about the current situation. Use good judgement when offering additional services. Make sure they have a clear understanding of what is being said to them. Address their immediate needs and concerns and continue your active listening. Your listening skills should include repeating back what they have shared with you, as well as acknowledgement of social cues like a nod of the head to let them know that they are being heard. In the event of a natural disaster, do not speculate on outcomes or make promises as to the safety of victims or those suffering in a mental health emergency. Reassure them using only the facts of the present moment and how you can assist.

KEEPING CALM AND SELF-REGULATING

When you or the other person are agitated, anxious or feel like you're losing control, know that you can change your arousal system and self-regulate to calm yourself down instantaneously. The following are some tried and true methods to help you get your emotions back under control in order to reach the level-headed state necessary to make decisions. You can either use these techniques yourself, as appropriate, or pass the information on to those you're helping.

Mindful Breathing

To quickly calm yourself in any situation, simply take 60 breaths, focusing your attention on each in-breath and each out-breath. Some people enjoy adding a mantra to this, where you focus on saying one word over and over during your breathing exercises.

For youths or adults, you may want to role-play "square breathing" with them. Take a deep breath for 5 seconds, hold for 5 seconds, breath out for 5 seconds, and rest for 5 seconds. Repeat a few times.

Another suggestion for younger children is diaphragmatic breathing. This method incorporates the person putting their hand on their diaphragm to feel the rise and fall of their lungs and chest with a slow, even cadence while they take a few deep breaths.

With any method you choose, please ensure the person is not breathing too rapidly, as this can cause dizziness.

Sensory Input

Just as certain smells or sounds can instantly transport you back in time to traumatic events (the sound of fireworks can bring a veteran right back into the combat zone, for example) so, too, can sensory input quickly calm you. Think back to a time when you felt happy, safe and at peace. What brought you that comfort? What can bring you back to that state? Looking at pictures of your loved ones, listening to a favorite song, reading a good book...everyone responds a little differently, so experiment to find what works best for you.

Reconnect Emotionally

By reconnecting to uncomfortable emotions in a controlled setting where you won't become overwhelmed, you can make a huge difference in your ability to manage stress, balance your moods, and take back control of the situation.

CHAPTER 20

De-Escalating a Situation

YOU AS THE first responder must take all warnings and threats seriously. If you are uncomfortable with a situation or are fearful for your own safety, seek help immediately. Never put yourself at risk. If a person's aggression and level of escalation is out of control, remove yourself immediately and call for emergency assistance. Remember to notify law enforcement regarding whether the person is armed or unarmed. If you are a law enforcement officer, please defer to your appropriate and professional training protocols.

AGGRESSION

Aggression is usually displayed in one of two forms:

1. Aggression that is driven by emotions and is based around fear, and

2. Aggression as a response to not getting the things that a person is used to getting

In the first case, the individual wants to be heard and understood, while in the second case, the individual wants an audience or a stage so that they can let their feelings explode.

When dealing with aggressive individuals, remain calm and stoic in your approach. Exercise empathy and your active listening skills, and re-direct the conversation with healthy, safe alternatives. Remember to keep your tactics simple.

If you have reason to believe the aggression is closely related to a mental health concern, call your local mental health crisis team or your medical oversight to assist you. If law enforcement officers are the only ones on the scene, it is important for you to advocate for the mental health of the individual in crisis, especially if you feel that a mental health concern or emergency is part of their aggressive behavior *and* that it can be reduced with proper mental health emergency tactics.

While you may now be in a position where you are equipped with more mental health information than ever before, please avoid diagnosing or "labeling" a person when reporting the events of an escalation to a professional. Keep your observations clear, concise and compact. Stick to using the descriptions you have learned, noting signs and symptoms of the behaviors that you have observed, in order to better aid the crisis workers who arrive on the scene.

DE-ESCALATING A SITUATION: THE BASICS

Aggressive behaviors need immediate attention and require swift intervention to prevent worsening of the symptoms and restore the safety of the situation at hand. A good de-escalation involves making sure you, your staff and the individual in distress are safe, and that you are exercising empathy through a calm and safe approach while providing a comfortable space that allows the person some room to breathe and to walk around or sit comfortably.

The idea is to quickly get into a rapport with the individual. Always be respectful, receptive and helpful to their sensitivities and needs. As you approach, provide your name, title and affiliation, and make sure your stance is comfortable, with legs shoulder-width apart, feet comfortably placed under your shoulders and arms opened comfortably. Provide a safe and clear distance from the individual that is one to two arm's-lengths away. Make sure your arms are uncrossed, hands unclenched. Keep your body language and economy of movement calm and your voice quiet, soothing and persuasive to subtly let them know you are in charge, as though to place someone at ease. Try not to exhibit facial expressions to the best of your ability. Make sure your legs are relaxed and knees are comfortably bent. Ensure that your body is not mirroring the individual straight on, and that you are slightly angled, as facing a person straight on can appear confrontational.

If they want more space and breathing room, give it to them. Tell them subtly that you are here to help. Make sure you have a proper method of exit if you are indoors, such as a doorway or window. Keep yourself close to the exit and give them plenty of room so they don't feel boxed in.

While you continue to engage and make verbal cues with the person, be clear and concise in your language. Concise language means using simple words. Keep your sentences short and your cadence slowly paced so the person has time to process what you are sharing with them. Often it is a good idea to repeat yourself until the person understands what you are trying to convey. Make the person understand that you both have boundaries, and try to offer simple safe choices and propose safe alternatives.

Do not belittle, criticize, trivialize or humiliate the person. Even if you've "been there before" and have had a similar experience, refrain from trivializing their experience. This includes any experiences common to young people which are currently distressing to that person. Refrain from comparing similar stories or making comments such as, "That's really not that bad." Use your good listening skills and acknowledge what the person is saying to you. Show empathy and find common ground with the person suffering.

Make sure you set boundaries up front. Let them know that you are in charge and that you will be understanding of their concerns and immediate needs. Remain positive in your approach and be able to provide options to that individual. Continue to check in and reassure the person.

Ask the individual what they want, using phrases like, "What is not working right now?" and "Please tell me if I'm understanding you correctly…" Note that you *are* allowed to disagree with the person, but try to empower them with positive information and motivate them by focusing on their positive qualities. Do not make promises that you cannot keep, but help the person to identify healthy, safe behavior that is not going to cause them or others harm or get them in trouble.

DE-ESCALATION TIPS AND TACTICS

When approaching a person in a mental health emergency to attempt to de-escalate the situation, here are some important things to remember:

- Stay calm, stoic, and keep relaxed and unflustered.

- Speak in a calm, soft, soothing, confident and succinct manner.

- Do not respond in a challenging, hostile or disciplinary manner; never argue or debate with the person! This will only complicate the situation.

- Do not threaten; this may escalate the situation and may increase fear, aggression and exacerbate their symptoms.

- Do not raise your voice or speak too quickly.

- Avoid using first responder speak, acronyms and medical jargon.

- Avoid using negative words; replace them with positive words.

- Be cognizant of your own body language, use economy of motion, and avoid any sudden movements or fidgeting.

- Do not restrict the person's movement; i.e., do not box them into a corner. If you are in an enclosed room, allow them to have an escape route. The same goes for yourself and your team members.

- Be mindful that involving law enforcement or emergency services may escalate the situation.

- Use breaks of silence to allow the person an opportunity to cool off. Remember, when in doubt as to what to say, use silence to your advantage.

- It is important to debrief your experience with the rest of your team to see what didn't work and what went well in your de-escalation techniques.

CHAPTER 21

Mental Health Self-Care

WHILE INFORMATION IS without a doubt your most powerful tool as a first responder, and having a clear understanding of the various types of illnesses, disorders and crises you may encounter is key, you cannot underestimate the need to practice proper self-care. While it's natural to think of your priority as being the other person's safety and well-being—after all, you're there to help them—placing yourself in an unsafe situation, or pushing yourself beyond your personal limits, doesn't do anybody any good.

In the following pages, we'll be discussing a few simple steps you can take to ensure that you stay completely focused and committed to the people you are helping.

THE IMPORTANCE OF SELF-CARE

The activities you engage in and the daily choices you make affect the way you feel and how much you're able to help yourself. These choices, in turn, affect those around you. Investing in self-care is as much about caring for others as it is for yourself.

Only when you feel healthy and happy can you be your smartest, most creative, most fit, and most caring self.

Some basic tips for practicing proper self-care include:

- **Getting enough rest.** To have good mental and emotional health, it's important to get enough sleep. Most people need about 7–8 hours of sleep each night. Make the investment in a better mattress.

- **Getting a dose of sunlight.** Sunlight lifts your mood, so try to get at least 10–15 minutes per day, or use a lightbox in winter or places that receive a lot less sunlight.

- **Enjoying the beauty of nature or art**. Simply walking can lower blood pressure and reduce stress. The same goes for walking through a park or an art gallery, hiking, or sitting on a beach.

- **Engaging in meaningful work.** Do things that challenge your creativity and make you feel productive, whether or not you get paid for it—things like marksmanship and martial arts competitions, advanced yoga classes, drawing, playing an instrument, or building something.

- **Getting a pet.** Pets are certainly a responsibility, but caring for one makes you feel needed and loved. Walking the dog can also be a great way to get you out of the house for exercise and expose you to new people and places.

- **Having fun!** Do things for no other reason than that it feels good to do them. Go to a comedy club, go for a hike, read a good book, or hangout with friends. Hard play is *not* an indulgence; it's a necessity for emotional and mental health.

- **Avoiding cigarettes, drugs and alcohol.** These stimulants make you feel unnaturally good in the short game, but have negative long-term game consequences for your mood and your emotional health.

- **Limiting screen time and tech neck.** We all love our smartphones and mobile devices but spending too much time staring at a screen denies you the face-to-face interactions that can meaningfully connect you to others.

- **Avoiding isolation.** Living alone or in a limited social circle due to relocation, aging, or decreased mobility can lead to isolation and an increased risk of depression. Whatever your situation, try to schedule regular social activities with friends, neighbors, colleagues, or family members who are upbeat, positive, and interested in you.

SUPPORT NETWORKS
FOR FIRST RESPONDERS

One of the key factors in improving mental/emotional health and building resilience is cultivating a support network. Having supportive people like friends and family around that you can talk to daily can have an overwhelmingly positive influence on your overall state of mental well-being. Humans are social creatures, with an overriding emotional need for relationships and positive connections with others. We're not meant to survive—let alone thrive—in isolation.

The key is to find a supportive relationship with someone who is a "good listener:" someone you can regularly talk to in person, who will listen to you without a pre-existing agenda for how you should think or feel. Face-to-face social interaction with someone who cares about you is the most effective way to calm your nervous system and relieve stress. Interacting with another person can quickly put the brakes on defensive stress responses, like "fight-or-flight," the term coined by Harvard Professor Walter Cannon in the 1920s, to describe an animal preparing to attack or flee during a perceived threat. He related this to how humans handle stress responses in similar fashion. By having someone to check in with, you gain the ability to release the hormones that reduce stress leading to you feeling better, even if you're unable to affect the stressful situation itself. A good listener will listen to the feelings *behind* your words. They won't interrupt, judge, or criticize you.

If you feel that you don't have anyone to turn to, there are good ways to build new friendships and improve your support network. To start with, get out from behind your TV or computer screen. Screens have their place, but so much of communication is nonverbal that a lack of direct contact with other people costs you the benefits of forging a real connection with others. Next, become a "joiner": join networking, social, or special interest groups that meet on a regular basis. These groups offer wonderful opportunities for meeting people with common interests. Remember, reaching out is *not* a sign of weakness, and it doesn't mean you're a burden to others. The truth is that most people are flattered when you trust them enough to confide in them.

STRESS RELIEF

So many of us spend most our daily lives feeling stressed, to the point that we're no longer even aware of it. Being stressed becomes our "normal." But when stress becomes overwhelming, it can damage your mood, trigger or aggravate mental and physical health problems, and affect the quality of your life.

The mind and the body are intrinsically linked. When you improve your physical health, you automatically experience greater mental and emotional well-being. Exercise is something you can engage in right now to boost your energy and outlook and help you regain a sense of control. Exercise not only strengthens your heart, lungs, and muscles; it also releases endorphins, powerful chemicals that lift your mood and provide added energy.

Regular exercise can have a positive impact on mental and emotional health problems, such as depression, bipolar disorder, anxiety, trauma, and attention deficit hyperactivity disorder (ADHD). Exercise also relieves stress, improves memory, and helps you to sleep better. And you don't have to be a fitness fanatic to reap the benefits—even modest amounts of exercise can make a big difference to your mental and emotional health. Aim for 30 minutes of activity on most days; or, if it's easier, three 10-minute sessions can be just as effective. Try rhythmic exercise that engages both your arms and legs, such as walking, running, swimming, weight training, martial arts, or dancing.

Better yet, add a mindfulness element to your workouts. Instead of focusing on your thoughts, focus on how your body feels as you move—how your feet hit the ground, the rhythm of your breathing, or the feeling of wind on your skin.

PROPER DIET AND NUTRITION

What you eat—and even more importantly, what you don't eat—has a direct impact on the way you feel. Wholesome meals give you more energy and help you look better, resulting in a boost to your self-esteem, while unhealthy food can take a massive toll on your brain, body and mood.

Our bodies respond differently to different foods, depending on our genetics and other health factors, so experiment to learn how the food you include in—or cut from—your diet affects the way you feel. In general, instead of obsessing over specific foods or nutrients, focus more on your overall eating pattern, how you take in certain foods and how the different varieties affect you.

Foods that adversely affect mood include:

- Caffeine: soda, coffee, and energy drinks

- Alcohol: beer, wine, grain alcohol, and sugary mixed cocktails

- Trans fats, or anything with "partially hydrogenated" oil

- Foods with high levels of chemical preservatives or hormones

- Sugary snacks

- Refined carbohydrates (such as white rice or white flour)

- Fried foods

Foods that boost mood include:

- Fatty fish rich in omega-3s, such as salmon, herring, mackerel, anchovies, sardines, and tuna. Be careful to eat certain fish in moderation as concerns over levels of mercury may adversely affect your physical health.

- Nuts, such as walnuts, almonds, cashews, peanuts

- Avocados

- Flaxseed

- Garlic, scallions and red onions

- Quinoa

- Beans

- Leafy greens, such as spinach, kale, Brussels sprouts

- Fresh fruit, such as blueberries and apples

- Dark chocolate

- Green tea

- Clean drinking water and hot water with lemon

SENSORY EXPERIENCES FOR STRESS RELIEF

While social interaction and exercise are both excellent ways to relieve stress, it's not always realistic to assume you'll have a friend close by to lean on when you feel stressed, or that you'll be able to go out for a run or a workout at the gym. The best way to reduce stress quickly and reliably is by just taking a deep breath and using your senses—what you see, hear, smell, taste, and touch—or soothing movement. By viewing a favorite photo, smelling a specific scent, listening to a favorite piece of music, tasting a piece of gum, or hugging a pet, for example, you can quickly relax and focus yourself.

Of course, not everyone responds to specific sensory experiences in the same way. What some people find soothing and relaxing may be unpleasant or even stressful to others. For example, certain kinds of music may relax and calm one person but do nothing but irritate someone else. So, to master quick stress relief techniques, you need to first become a "stress-busting first responder," and track down the sensory experiences that effectively and efficiently make you calm and alert.

First, understand that there is a difference between sensory experiences that are pleasant, those that are intense, and those that are enjoyable enough to quickly make you feel both calm and alert. In the time it takes you to pet your dog, recall a few lines of your favorite song, or taste the sensation of licking ice cream or biting into a piece of dark chocolate, you should begin to feel your stress begin to ease, your head start to clear, and your sense of control returning. If it takes you an entire yoga class, half a dozen cups of tea and several hours of meditation to regain your wellness, try something else. If the effect is too subtle, keep investigating what sensory experiences put you at ease.

Each time you feel stressed, try a different sensory experience and note how long it takes for your stress levels drop. Remember: you're looking for something that works almost immediately. As you experiment, be as precise as possible. What is the most perfect image, the specific kind of sound, or type of movement that affects you the most? For example, if you're a music lover, listen to many different artists and types of music until you find a jam that instantly makes you feel more in control of yourself just by thinking of it.

Use the following examples as your frame of reference. Give your imagination free rein and come up with additional sensory experiences to try.

Sight

If you're a visual person, try to relieve stress by surrounding yourself with soothing and uplifting images. If there's nothing within eyesight, try closing your eyes, taking a deep breath, and imagining a soothing image. Another idea would be to create a vision board on your refrigerator with all your dreams and goals laid out in stunning photos.

- Keep a cherished photo on your phone, mobile device or in your wallet, be it of your child, your pet, a fun night out with friends, or an image from a memorable vacation.

- Watch a relaxing desktop screensaver or YouTube videos with soothing, uplifting images and music.

- Try widening your vision. Begin with a single focus and, with each breath or blink, try to widen your field by a few objects until you have full vision (including peripheral).

- If you have a pleasant view from your home or office window, spend a few moments gazing outside. If movement relaxes you, choose chairs that are movable like a rocking chair and rock back in forth.

Touch

Experiment with your sense of touch, playing with different tactile sensations of the body.

- Try curling your toes, tensing your feet and tensing body parts all the way up your spine to the crown of your head.

- Try placing a rubber band around your wrist. This can act as a cue to remind you to check in with yourself. When you feel stressed, gently snap the band and use the best sensory tools available to relax.

- Pet a dog or cat, or hug a friend. It can lower your blood pressure and dissolve the stress away.

- Squeeze a stress ball or clap your hands. Drum your hands to the beat of one of your favorite songs.

- Squeeze your fingers and watch your circulation.

- If a piece of ice is handy, hold it for a ten seconds, feeling the sensations as it calms your whole body.

- Wear clothing that feels good against your skin, like cottons or silks.

Taste

Taking the time to slowly savor a favorite treat like chocolate, ice cream or nuts can be very relaxing, but mindless eating will only add to your stress levels and concerns about your health. The key is to indulge your sense of taste mindfully and in moderation. Eat slowly, focusing on the feel of the food in your mouth and the taste on your tongue.

- Chewing a piece of gum can lower levels of the stress hormone cortisol.

- Indulge in small pieces of dark chocolate or healthy snacks like nuts.

- When you feel yourself dissociate, grab a piece of hard candy with a strong taste, be it sour or spicy. This can quickly engage your senses and allow you to ground yourself and begin the process of checking in with yourself.

- Take a bite of a ripe piece of fruit, like a mango or pineapple, for a taste of the tropics.

- Swallow a few mouthfuls of your favorite tea or coffee. Make sure to go easy on the coffee, as it is known to induce anxiety.

- Keep crunchy snacks like celery, carrots, or trail mix nearby.

Movement

If you tend to shut down when you're under stress or have experienced trauma, stress-relieving activities that get you moving may be particularly helpful. Shut down (also known as disassociation) is experienced as an unbidden interruption of one's awareness and behavior, along with accompanying losses of continuity and subjective experience (i.e., "positive" dissociative symptoms such as fragmentation of identity, depersonalization, and derealization). It can also lead to an inability to access information or to control mental functions that normally are readily amenable to access or control (i.e., "negative" dissociative symptoms such as amnesia).

When your stress levels are high and you feel that you are dissociating, it is imperative you stay focused and in the moment. It may be necessary to take a few of the steps simultaneously to become fully aware of your surroundings and begin a self-check in.

- Briefly step outside. Walk around the block and savor the sunshine (or the rain).

- Repetitive motions like brushing your hair or knitting can help you relax.

- Bounce or tap your heels.

- Stretch or roll your head in circles.

- Sit on something you can bounce on.

LEARNING TO USE YOUR SENSES AS A FIRST RESPONDER

It's not easy to remember to use your senses in the middle of a mini—or not so mini—crisis. At first, it will feel easier to just give into pressure and tense up. But with time—and lots of practice—calling upon your senses when you're stressed will become second nature.

Learning to use your senses to quickly manage stress is a little like learning to drive or play golf. You don't master the skill in one lesson; you must practice. Once you have a variety of sensory tools you can depend on, you'll be able to handle even the toughest of situations.

Here are some tips to help you make quick stress relief a habit:

- **Start small.** Instead of testing your quick stress relief tools on a source of major stress, start with a predictable low-level source of stress, like cooking dinner at the end of the day, washing dishes or organizing your work papers.

- **Identify and target.** Think of just one low-level stressor that you know will occur several times a week, such as the commute to work. Vow to target that stressor with quick stress relief every time. Practice mindfulness actives when you are stuck in traffic. After a few weeks, target a second stressor. After a few weeks, target a second and third stressor, and so on.

- **Test-drive sensory input.** Experiment with as much sensory input as possible. For example, if you are practicing quick stress relief on your commute to work, bring a scented handkerchief with you one day, try music another day, and then try sucking a mint the next day.

- **Don't force it.** If something doesn't work, move on until you find your best fit.

- **Talk about it.** Verbalizing your quick stress relief experiments will help you integrate it into your life. It's bound to start a long-winded conversation with colleagues, friends and family—everyone relates to the topic of stress.

- **Journaling. Try using a simple diary to keep track of your progress.**

Becoming adept at quick stress relief will help you successfully navigate stressful situations. It will also be an invaluable aid in learning the type of meditation that fosters social and emotional connection.

CONCLUSION

Thank you for taking an interest in mental health, and for picking up *Mental Health Emergencies: A First Responder's Guide to Recognizing and Handling Crises.* Our hope is that this book has helped you learn to identify the risks and warning signs concerning mental health and substance use issues. The content and tactics provided here are ones you can take to aid, assist, or even save someone's life. You may find yourself preventing the act of an overdose or stopping someone that is actively self-injuring, or even suicidal. While this newfound knowledge may increase your confidence, please make sure to refer to the text often to keep your first responder skills fresh. In addition, consider pursuing training courses and other official certifications to make the best use of your mental health literacy and skills.

As you continue your journey, you will begin to help demystify stigmas, empowering and encouraging others with your new heightened awareness, and communicating and listening in an empathetic manner. The important strategies you have learned are meant to help someone in and out of crises. This includes taking care of your own mental health using the self-care hacks included in this book.

As a first responder, always remember that assistance should be given until the mental health emergency resolves, or until the appropriate medical or mental health professionals arrive on the scene to assist in the next steps of treatment.

We recommend you tell your colleagues, friends, families, and anyone you may encounter about *Mental Health Emergen-*

cies: A First Responder's Guide to Recognizing and Handling Crises, and encourage them to go out and receive formal training and certification in the field of mental health. Please remember: you play an important role in people's lives, and being prepared for an emergency can help save lives.

So please, help spread the word!

As a first responder, with the aid of this guide, you should now be able to:

1. Understand the need for proper training as it applies to mental health concerns, crises and emergencies.

2. Be able to break stigmas and dispel misconceptions of mental health with your colleagues and peers.

3. Learn how to work with sensitive and vulnerable mental health populations.

4. Learn first responder-based interactions with the mentally ill using tactics drawn from Behavioral Health Units (BHU) and evidence-based models and practices.

5. Clearly understand and describe the difference between basic mental health emergency assistance and professional medical and mental help.

6. Identify common personality traits and mental health disorders that may or may not be confused with physical ailments on emergency calls.

7. Use this resource as a supplement to your existing protocols, but not as a replacement.

8. Clearly define behavioral impairments such as anxiety, depression, grief, panic, mania, suicidal ideations and self-injurious behavior.

9. Prevent yourself from fatigue and burnout.

10. Assist, document and archive for hospital pre-screenings/histories.

11. Operate during mass casualty and traumatic events and use your mental health knowledge tactically.

12. Deter media attention and aid and assist any bystanders, friends and family members.

13. Use role playing scripts.

14. Develop and hone your active listening skills, empathy and emotional intelligence toolkit by reading body language and social clues.

15. Employ de-escalation techniques to minimize potentially aggressive and violent encounters, while increasing the overall safety of the scene.

16. Be persistent with seeking help. Do not give up; continue seeking assistance until you feel satisfied the person in the mental health emergency will receive the proper care.

RESOURCES

American Psychiatric Association
Web: https://www.psychiatry.org
(888) 35-PSYCH or (888) 357-7924
(703) 907-7300 for callers from outside the U.S. and Canada

National Center for Child Traumatic Stress (NCCTS)
NCCTS — University of California, Los Angeles
11150 W. Olympic Blvd., Suite 650
Los Angeles, CA 90064
Phone: (310) 235-2633
Fax: (310) 235-2612

NCCTS — Duke University
1121 West Chapel Hill Street Suite 201
Durham, NC 27701
Phone: (919) 682-1552
Fax: (919) 613-9898

Program Office of the National Child Traumatic Stress Initiative; Center for Mental Health Services; Substance Abuse and Mental Health Services Administration; Department of Health and Human Services
5600 Fishers Lane
Parklawn Building, Room 17C-26
Rockville, MD 20857

Mental Health First Aid USA

www.mentalhealthfirstaid.org

Mental Health First Aid Australia

www.mhfa.com.au

Developed in 2000 by Betty Kitchener, AM, and Professor Tony Jorm, Mental Health First Aid Australia is a national not-for-profit organization focused on mental health training and research. MHFA Australia develops, evaluates and provides a variety of training programs and courses, including evidence-based MHFA courses, which teach mental health first aid strategies to members of the public, and instructor training courses, which train and accredit suitable individuals to deliver these MHFA courses to communities and workplaces across Australia.

National Institute of Mental Health

Prevalence of Mental Disorders in America

www.nimh.nih.gov

The National Institute of Mental Health website provides statistics pertaining to mental disorders, including prevalence data by age, sex, race, and average age of onset.

National Council for Community Behavioral Healthcare

www.thenationalcouncil.org

Contact them to locate mental health and addictions treatment facilities in your community.

Veteran Mental Health Resources

www.mentalhealth.va.gov

National Alliance on Mental Illness (NAMI)

www.nami.org

The nation's largest grassroots mental health organization dedicated to building better lives for the millions of Americans affected by mental illness, NAMI started as a small group of families gathered around a kitchen table in 1979 and has blossomed into the nation's leading voice on mental health. Today, NAMI is an association of hundreds of local affiliates, state organizations and volunteers who work in your community to raise awareness and provide support and education that was not previously available to those in need.

CALL THE NAMI HELPLINE
Phone: 800-950-NAMI
Email: info@nami.org
Monday–Friday, 10 AM–6 PM ET
Find help in a crisis or text "NAMI" to 741741

Mental Health America

www.mentalhealthamerica.net

Mental Health America's site gathers information on mental health, and provides tips on how to get help and take action. Call toll-free: 1-800-969-6642

HELP LINES

National Suicide Prevention Lifeline

1-800-273-TALK (8255)

- 24 hours a day
- Free and confidential
- Trained counselors
- Veterans services

Veterans Crisis Line
www.veteranscrisisline.net
1-800-273-8255

American Psychological Association Public Education Line
1-800-964-2000
Follow the operator's instructions to be connected to a professional.

The Trevor Project
This is a free and confidential suicide prevention help line for gay and questioning youths that offers hope and an outlet to speak to someone, 24 hours a day.
PO Box 69232
West Hollywood, CA 90069
info@thetrevorproject.org
Phone: 310-271-8845

American Psychiatric Association Answer Center
Phone: 1-888-35-PSYCH (77924)
Operators can refer you to local board certified psychiatrists.

Anxiety Disorders Resource Center
www.anxietypanickattack.com
Information on panic attacks, generalized anxiety, social anxiety, depression, obsessive-compulsive disorder, and post-traumatic stress disorder.

Something Fishy
www.somethingfishy.org
Useful information for those affected with eating disorders. Great place to find support groups.

Overeaters Anonymous

www.oa.org
Helps individuals struggling with compulsive and binge
eating.

National Eating Disorders Association

www.nationaleatingdisorders.org

National Association of Anorexia Nervosa and Associated Disorders

www.anad.org

Obsessive-Compulsive Foundation

www.ocfoundation.org
Find information on obsessive compulsive-disorder and effective treatments.

Families for Depression Awareness

www.familyaware.org
391 Totten Pond Road, Suite 101
Waltham, MA 02451
Telephone: 781-890-0220 (main office) or 615-345-0420
(satellite office in Nashville, TN)
Fax: 781-890-2411
Email: info@familyaware.org

Depression and Bipolar Support Alliance (DBSA)

www.dbsalliance.org
Phone: 1-800-826-3632

Early Assessment and Support Alliance

www.easacommunity.org

A great resource for young people who have experienced psychosis.

EASA Technical Assistance Team

To contact the EASA technical assistance team, please use the following contact information:

Regional Research Institute (RRI)

Portland State University

Suite 900

1600 SW 4th Ave.

Portland OR 97201

SARDAA | "Shattering Stigma-Realizing Recovery"

Schizophrenia and Related Disorders Alliance of America

PO Box 941222

Houston, TX 77094-8222

Phone: 240-423-9432

800-493-2094 (toll-free)

Email: info@sardaa.org

Mayo Clinic

www.mayoclinic.org

Mayo Clinic is a nonprofit organization committed to clinical practice, education and research, providing expert, whole-person care to everyone who needs healing.

Resources for LGBTIQ

www.samhsa.gov

Schizophrenia.com

Started in 1995, Schizophrenia.com is a leading community

dedicated to providing high quality information, support and education to the family members, caregivers and individuals whose lives have been impacted by schizophrenia.

POLITICAL RESOURCES

The Honorable Patrick J. Kennedy, former member of the U.S. House of Representatives

www.patrickjkennedy.net

Visit their website to find out more about Patrick and his wife's initiatives regarding mental health and addictions.

The Kennedy Forum

www.thekennedyforum.org

Receive updates on legal, medical and scientific news; a great resource for driving solutions for mental health and addictions.

One Mind

www.onemind.org

An open forum for big data, science and advanced collaboration in brain research.

SAM: Smart Approaches to Marijuana

www.learnaboutsam.org

Health-first approach to marijuana policy.

ParityTrack.Org

www.paritytrack.org

Collaboration between the Kennedy Forum, the Thomas Scattergood Foundation and the Treatment Research Institute, ParityTrack.org helps implement and enforce the 2008 Mental Health Parity and Addiction Equity Act.

ABOUT THE AUTHORS

Nick Benas, QMHA (Qualified Mental Health Associate) is a former United States Marine Sergeant and Iraqi Combat Veteran. Nick is the former Director of Business Operations for Clatsop Behavioral Healthcare, a private non-profit mental health agency, located on the Columbia River in Astoria, Oregon. He is also a Certified Mental Health First Aid Instructor by the National Council for Behavioral Health, teaching adults, and youth modules. He travels around the United States training individuals on how to recognize a developing mental illness and how to prevent someone from slipping into a crisis. He has been featured by more than 50 major media outlets for his business success and entrepreneurship, including Entrepreneur Magazine, Men's Health, ABC, FOX, ESPN, and CNBC.

Michele Hart, LCSW is Licensed Clinical Social Worker in the State of Utah with over 20 years' experience in the field of social work. Throughout her career, she has worked in a variety of settings including residential and outpatient clinics, educational settings and probation and parole. Her primary focus and passion has been centered around trauma and its impact on children, families and adults. Michele's clinical background has been providing individual and group services as both a therapist and a Clinical Director. She utilizes best practices models of Cognitive Behavioral Therapy, Trauma Competency and Motivational Interviewing to provide diagnosis and treatment of:

- Trauma and stressor related disorders
- Anxiety disorders
- Depressive disorders
- Obsessive-compulsive and related disorders
- Bipolar and related disorders
- Schizophrenia spectrum and other psychotic disorders

GLOSSARY OF TERMS

Abandonment: when a person suffering with a mental health concern or crisis is left alone by a first responder or professional and/or left to the care of someone who is not equipped to provide proper support

Abdominal breathing: a technique that utilizes breaths from the diaphragm (breathing from the belly region)

Acclimatization: when an individual physiologically adjusts to an environment

Acute: mental health condition(s) that need immediate attention; these are often sudden and unexpected

Advanced directive: a legally binding document, usually included in a living will or a power of attorney, which dictates the direction of one's own medical and mental healthcare if they are not able to advocate for their own healthcare needs

Affect: term that refers to emotion and state of emotion. "Flat affect" refers to having little or no signs of emotion; i.e., there's no relationship between the emotion a person is feeling and what they are thinking.

Aggression: explosive, violent and hostile behavior

Agoraphobia: anxiety around places or situations; the fear of having a panic attack when away from home, especially in large crowded public spaces.

Alogia: diminished speech output

Alzheimer's disease: a type of dementia that becomes progressively worse; most prevalent in people 65 years of age and older.

Ambiguity: having multiple meanings

Ambivalence: indecision on how one feels; the person experiences conflict between feelings that are often mutually incompatible

Ambulatory: the person in crisis is able to walk to a safe, quiet location

Amnesia: when a person has loss of memory

Anhedonia: the inability to experience pleasure from positive stimuli or degradation in the recollection of pleasure from previous events

Anomia: the inability of a person to remember names

Anorexia nervosa: extreme weight-loss strategies used to control body weight; includes: dieting, fasting, hyper-exercise, slimming pills, diuretics, laxatives and vomiting

Antipsychotic drugs: medications designed to alleviate the symptoms of mental illness and assist with the treatment of psychosis

Anxiety: feelings of uneasiness and tension based around a perceived threat. Often the person does not know why their "fight or flight" alarm system is responding.

Asociality: a lack of interest in social interactions

Attention Deficit Disorder/Attention Deficit Hyperactivity Disorder (ADD/ADHD): persistent and uncontrollable inattention, distractibility, and restlessness

Attitude: a person's learned response to other people and events

Auscultation: the action of listening to an individual's heart and lungs with a stethoscope during a quick medical screening

Autism: a rare brain disorder, usually discovered in infancy; symptoms include emotional detachment, the inability to relate to others, abnormality in speech and communication, and an unusually high level of interest in objects or things

Avolition: a decrease in motivated self-initiated activities. A person may just sit for long periods of time and show little interest in participating in work or social activities.

Bipolar disorder: once commonly referred to as manic-depressive disorder, it is a mood disorder where serious episodes of depression ("lows") alternate with serious episodes of mania (or extreme "highs")

Bulimia nervosa: frequent and recurring episodes of eating unusually large amounts of food and a lack of control over eating, followed by purging, fasting and hyper-exercise

Catatonia: describes a condition in which the person is withdrawn, in an unresponsive state, and exhibits strange body language/movements, usually accompanied by a refusal to move

Chronic: the opposite of acute; describes a condition that is continuous, or reoccurring over extended periods of time; in the case of mental health, it can be used to indicate that a condition is severe and persistent, or that the symptoms may recur occasionally

Commitment: in mental health, an involuntary hospitalization that requires a legal procedure in which professionals must provide evidence of mental illness, the inability to care for one's self and the potential for danger to themselves or others

Competency: ability to make decisions that safely impact the person you're helping in a mental health emergency

Compulsion: an urge to engage in and perform a certain behavior

Co-morbidity: existing simultaneously with, and usually independently of, another medical condition

Conduct Disorder: language applied to youth and adolescents when describing persistent patterns of behaviors that impact one's quality of life

CSM: circulation, sensation, motion

Delusion: a false idea, misconstruction, or strange idea not usually accepted by others

Dementia: a condition of memory loss, cognitive deficit, and a difficulty in learning new information, as well as a loss of mental abilities the individual once had

Depression: described often as the "black hole" or "fog of war," a constant feeling of impending doom, and feelings of sadness and hopelessness

Diminished Emotional Expression: reductions in the expression of emotions in the face, eye contact, speech and movement of the hand, head and face that normally give emotional emphasis to speech

DNR: abbreviation for "do not resuscitate;" a written advance directive not to resuscitate in the event the person is in cardiac arrest

Dysthymic Disorder: from the Greek term dysthymia, meaning "ill humor" or "bad mood"

Eating Disorder(s): serious, life-threatening mental illnesses involving eating habits, purging and body image

ETOH: a medical term for an individual suffering with alcohol use

Euphoria: elated, having an elevated or high mood state

Fight or Flight: a person's response to stress to stay and fight or run away

First Responder: someone designated, trained and equipped to respond to a mental health emergency

Genetic: referring to genes, the "blueprints" for traits passed from parents to their children through the sperm and egg cells; some traits are at risk for developing certain mental illnesses

Good Samaritan Laws: laws that encourage citizens to act in good faith to aid and assist during a medical or mental health crisis or emergency. Its intention is to minimize the risk and liability of the first responder if they are acting in good faith.

Grief: an emotional response to loss

Gross Negligence: when a first responder or professional deviates from the appropriate and accepted level of care

Hallucination: a false experience of senses; a perception of something that is not present. These are very real to the person experiencing them, and as a first responder you should validate the person's observations and not try to disprove their findings.

HR: heart rate

Hypertension: high blood pressure

Hyperventilation: rapid, deep breathing that usually occurs as a result of anxiousness or sudden and unexpected panic attacks

Informed Consent: when an individual who is suffering from a mental health emergency is informed of appropriate professional medical supports

Mania: great excitement, marked with "highs," euphoria and over-activity

Mental Health Advisor: a licensed mental health professional that advises a practitioner, first responder and/or working professionals

MHE: stands for Mental Health Emergency

Mood: a temporary state of mind or feeling

Mood Disorders: a psychological disorder characterized by the elevation or lowering of one's mood

MHX: shorthand for mental health history

Negligence: an unintentional act that harms an individual under duty of care

Obsession: a persistent idea, thought, image or impulse that consumes a person, often resulting in unhealthy or compulsive behaviors

Obsessive Compulsive Disorder (OCD): a disorder that includes uncontrollable obsessive thoughts and compulsive behaviors

Palpate: to feel by touching

Panic Attack: a sudden overwhelming feeling of disabling fear and anxiety

Paranoia: intense anxious and fearful feelings centered around perceived threats, persecution and conspiracy; may manifest as an extreme suspiciousness of people and events

Phobia: excessive, unreasonable fear of specific situations or objects

Psychiatrist: a medical doctor who has received specialty training in mental health; they are able to diagnose and treat, as well as administer medications

Psychologist: a mental health professional who has received a graduate degree in psychology, certified to do psychological testing and psychotherapy

Psychosis: a mental health problem in which a person has lost some contact with reality, resulting in severe disturbances in emotion, thinking and behavior

Psychotherapy: a general term for treating mental health by talking with a psychiatrist, psychologist or other mental health professional

Psychotic: a person suffering from a psychosis

Rx: shorthand for medication prescription, often seen on pill bottles.

Self-Injury: harming one's self by burning skin, cutting and slitting wrists, pulling, and plucking hair

Social Health: a term used interchangeably with emotional intelligence, emotional and physical health

Somatic Symptoms: describes a scenario in which an individual has a strong focus on their physical symptoms by way of anxiety, shown through excessive thoughts, feelings, and behaviors that relate to the physical symptoms that they are experiencing. These create a great amount of distress, which becomes a major disruption in their quality of life.

Standard of Care: the high level of professionalism a first responder exhibits when administering help in a mental health emergency

Suicide: when some attempts to take their own life; a completed suicide's end result is death

Tx: shorthand for treatment

SELECTED BIBLIOGRAPHY

What Are Personality Disorders? (n.d.) 2017
psychiatry.org/patients-families/personality-disorders/what-are-personality-disorders?_ga=1.84782105.1484572156.1488
644703

What Is Depression? (n.d.). 2017
www.psychiatry.org/patients-families/depression/what-is-depression?_ga=1.118328329.1484572156.1488644703

EASA Early Assessment and Support Alliance. (n.d.)
What is Psychosis? 2017
www.easacommunity.org/what-is-psychosis.php

The Fool's Tower. (n.d.) 2017
www.viennadirect.com/sights/hospital.php

About Schizophrenia. (n.d.) 2017
www.sardaa.org/resources/about-schizophrenia/

Schizophrenia and children and offspring. (n.d.)
schizophrenia.com/family/FAQoffspring.htm

Kitchener BA, and Jorm AF, Kelly CM
Mental Health First Aid Australia www.mhfa.com.au

Kitchener BA, and Jorm AF (2002)
Mental Health First Aid Manual
ORYGEN Research Centre, Melbourne, Australia
(Reprinted with amendments, 2008)

Kitchener BA, Jorm AF, Kelly CM
Youth Mental Health First Aid Manual, 2nd ed.
Melbourne: Mental Health First Aid Australia; 2010.

Forsyth MD, Hyde MO
Know About Mental Illness
New York: 1996

Koocher GP, La Greca AM
The Parents' Guide to Psychological First Aid
Oxford: 2011

American Psychiatric Association (2013)
Diagnostic and statistical manual of mental disorders: DSM-5
Washington, DC: American Psychiatric Association

Notes

Notes

Notes

Notes

Notes

Notes

Notes

Notes